Healthcare Associated Infections in the Neonatal Intensive Care Unit

Guest Editors

KAREN D. FAIRCHILD, MD
RICHARD A. POLIN, MD

CLINICS IN PERINATOLOGY

www.perinatology.theclinics.com

September 2010 • Volume 37 • Number 3

SAUNDERS an imprint of ELSEVIER, Inc.

W.B. SAUNDERS COMPANY
A Division of Elsevier Inc.

Elsevier, Inc. • 1600 John F. Kennedy Blvd. • Suite 1800 • Philadelphia, PA 19103-2899

http://www.theclinics.com

CLINICS IN PERINATOLOGY Volume 37, Number 3
September 2010 ISSN 0095-5108, ISBN-13: 978-1-4377-2479-0

Editor: Carla Holloway
Developmental Editor: Donald Mumford

Clinics in Perinatology (ISSN 0095-5108) is published quarterly by Elsevier Inc., 360 Park Avenue South, New York, NY 10010-1710. Months of issue are March, June, September, and December. Business and Editorial Offices: 1600 John F. Kennedy Blvd., Ste. 1800, Philadelphia, PA 19103-2899. Customer Service Office: 3251 Riverport Lane, Maryland Heights, MO 63043. Periodicals postage paid at New York, NY and additional mailing offices. Subscription prices are $239.00 per year (US individuals), $347.00 per year (US institutions), $281.00 per year (Canadian individuals), $441.00 per year (Canadian institutions), $345.00 per year (foreign individuals), $441.00 per year (foreign institutions) $116.00 per year (US students), and $168.00 per year (Canadian and foreign students). Foreign air speed delivery is included in all Clinics subscription prices. All prices are subject to change without notice. **POSTMASTER:** Send address changes to *Clinics in Perinatology*, Elsevier Health Sciences Division, Subscription Customer Service, 3251 Riverport Lane, Maryland Heights, MO 63043. **Customer Service: Telephone: 1-800-654-2452** (U.S. and Canada); **1-314-447-8871** (outside U.S. and Canada). **Fax: 1-314-447-8029. E-mail: journalscustomerservice-usa@elsevier.com** (for print support); **journalsonlinesupport-usa@elsevier.com** (for online support).

Reprints. For copies of 100 or more, of articles in this publication, please contact the Commercial Reprints Department, Elsevier Inc., 360 Park Avenue South, New York, NY 10010-1710. Tel. (212) 633-3812; Fax: (212) 482-1935; email: reprints@elsevier.com.

Clinics in Perinatology is also pubilshed in Spanish by McGraw-Hill Interamericana Editores S.A., P.O. Box 5-237, 06500 Mexico D.F., Mexico.

Clinics in Perinatology is covered in *MEDLINE/PubMed (Index Medicus) Current Contents, Excepta Medica, BIOSIS and ISI/BIOMED.*

Printed in the United States of America.

Contributors

GUEST EDITORS

KAREN D. FAIRCHILD, MD
Associate Professor of Pediatrics, Division of Neonatology, University of Virginia Hospital, Charlottesville, Virginia

RICHARD A. POLIN, MD
Professor of Pediatrics; Vice Chairman for Clinical and Academic Affairs, Department of Pediatrics; Director, Division of Neonatology, College of Physicians and Surgeons, Columbia University; Morgan Stanley Children's Hospital of New York, New York, New York

AUTHORS

ALISON J. CAREY, MD
Assistant Professor of Pediatrics, Drexel University College of Medicine; Attending Physician, Division of Neonatology, St. Christopher's Hospital for Children, Philadelphia, Pennsylvania

KAREN D. FAIRCHILD, MD
Associate Professor of Pediatrics, Division of Neonatology, University of Virginia, Charlottesville, Virginia

JEFFERY S. GARLAND, MD, SM
Department of Pediatrics, Wheaton Franciscan Healthcare, St. Joseph Hospital; Clinical Associate Professor, Department of Pediatrics, Medical College of Wisconsin; Clinical Associate Professor, Department of Pediatrics, University of Wisconsin School of Medicine and Public Health, Milwaukee, Wisconsin

PHILIP L. GRAHAM III, MD, MSc
Assistant Professor of Pediatrics, Division of Pediatric Infectious Diseases, Columbia University College of Physicians and Surgeons; Adjunct Assistant of Pediatrics, Weill Cornell Medical College; Hospital Epidemiologist/Quality and Patient Safety Officer, Department of Infection Prevention and Control, Division of Quality and Patient Safety, New York-Presbyterian Hospital, New York, New York

DENIS GRANDGIRARD, PhD
Senior Research Fellow, Neuro-Infectiology Laboratory, Institute for Infectious Diseases, University of Bern, Bern, Switzerland

DAVID A. KAUFMAN, MD
Associate Professor of Pediatrics, Division of Neonatology, Department of Pediatrics, University of Virginia School of Medicine, Charlottesville, Virginia

HUGH S. LAM, MRCPCH
Department of Pediatrics, Prince of Wales Hospital, The Chinese University of Hong Kong, Hong Kong

STEPHEN L. LEIB, MD
Associate Professor, Head, Neuro-Infectiology Laboratory, Institute for Infectious Diseases, University of Bern; Attending Physician, Clinic for Infectious Diseases, University Hospital, Bern, Switzerland

SARAH S. LONG, MD
Professor of Pediatrics, Drexel University College of Medicine; Chief, Division of Infectious Diseases, St. Christopher's Hospital for Children, Philadelphia, Pennsylvania

PAOLO MANZONI, MD
Neonatology and NICU, S. Anna Hospital, Torino, Italy

PAK C. NG, MD, FRCPCH
Department of Pediatrics, Prince of Wales Hospital, The Chinese University of Hong Kong, Hong Kong

T. MICHAEL O'SHEA, MD
Professor of Pediatrics, Chief, Division of Neonatology, Wake Forest University, Winston-Salem, North Carolina

SAMEER J. PATEL, MD
Assistant Professor of Pediatrics, Department of Pediatrics, Columbia University, New York, New York

TARA M. RANDIS, MD
Assistant Professor of Pediatrics, Division of Neonatology, Columbia University Medical Center, New York, New York

LISA SAIMAN, MD, MPH
Professor of Clinical Pediatrics, Department of Pediatrics, Columbia University; Hospital Epidemiologist, Department of Infection Prevention and Control, Morgan Stanley Children's Hospital of New York-Presbyterian, New York, New York

MICHAEL P. SHERMAN, MD
Professor of Child Health, Director, Neonatology Fellowship Program, University of Missouri, Columbia, Missouri

Contents

> *Staphylococcus aureus* is a continuously evolving and formidable patho-
> gen that has been a problem for both healthy and sick neonates for
> decades. Much focus over the past 20 years has been on hospital-associ-
> ated methicillinresistant *S aureus* (HA-MRSA); however, a global epidemic
> because of virulent community-associated MRSA (CA-MRSA) that has no
> "fitness cost" for carrying antibiotic-resistance genes has moved into neo-
> natal intensive care units (NICUs). Recently, methicillin-susceptible
> *S aureus* has adopted some of the virulence factors of CA-MRSA and is
> an increasingly common cause of hospital-acquired infections in NICUs.
> This article reviews the changing epidemiology, clinical manifestations,
> and treatment of *S aureus* in neonates.

> Antimicrobial-resistant pathogens are of increasing concern in the neona-
> tal intensive care unit population. A myriad of resistance mechanisms exist
> in microorganisms, and management can be complex because broad-
> spectrum antibiotics are increasingly needed. Control and prevention
> of antibiotic-resistant organisms (AROs) require an interdisciplinary team
> with continual surveillance. Judicious use of antibiotics; minimizing expo-
> sure to risk factors, when feasible; and effective hand hygiene are crucial
> interventions to reduce infection and transmission of AROs.

> Bacterial translocation from the gastrointestinal tract is an important path-
> way initiating late-onset sepsis and necrotizing enterocolitis in very low-
> birth-weight infants. The emerging intestinal microbiota, nascent intestinal
> epithelia, naive immunity, and suboptimal nutrition (lack of breast milk)
> have roles in facilitating bacterial translocation. Feeding lactoferrin, probi-
> otics, or prebiotics has presented exciting possibilities to prevent bacterial
> translocation in preterm infants, and clinical trials will identify the most safe
> and efficacious prevention and treatment strategies.

Early detection of late-onset neonatal sepsis, before the onset of obvious and potentially catastrophic clinical signs, is an important goal in neonatal medicine. Sepsis causes a well-known series of physiologic changes including abnormalities of blood pressure, respiration, temperature, and heart rate, and less well-known changes in heart rate variability. Although vital signs are frequently or continuously monitored in patients in the neonatal intensive care unit (NICU), changes in these parameters are subtle in the early phase of sepsis and difficult to interpret using traditional NICU monitoring tools. A new tool, continuous monitoring of heart rate characteristics (HRC), is now available for clinical use. Recent research has established that 2 abnormalities of HRC that have long been used by obstetricians to identify fetal compromise, reduced heart rate variability and transient decelerations, occur early in the course of sepsis in patients in the NICU, often before clinical signs of illness. Through mathematical modeling of electrocardiogram data from hundreds of patients in the NICU, an HRC index that represents the fold increase in risk that a neonate will be diagnosed with clinical or culture-proven sepsis within the next 24 hours was derived. The effect of continuous HRC monitoring on outcomes in preterm very low birth weight infants is the subject of a multicenter randomized clinical trial of 3000 patients, which will be complete in 2010. Further research into mechanisms of abnormal HRC and regulation of autonomic nervous system function in sepsis and other disease processes will shed light on additional applications of this exciting new technology.

Acute phase reactants, pro and antiinflammatory mediators including chemokines and cytokines, and cell-surface antigens are nonspecific biomarkers that have been extensively studied for the diagnosis and management of late-onset neonatal sepsis (LONS) and necrotizing enterocolitis. It is expected that the next generation of biomarkers and tests will be more specific, will pinpoint the precise disease entity, and will provide crucial information on the exact pathogen or category of microorganism and its antibiotic profile within hours of clinical presentation. Research on molecular pathogen detection and proteomic profiling has shown promising results. Academic-industry partnerships are vital for successful development of new diagnostic biomarkers for LONS, which are sensitive, inexpensive, fully automated, and easy to measure, allowing a quick turnaround time for clinical decision making.

The highest incidence of invasive candidal infection (ICI) occurs in extremely preterm infants (<1000 g birth weight and ≤27 weeks' gestation). In this population, ICI has high mortality, leads to significant neurodevelopmental impairment, and results in increased length of hospital stay and costs. Randomized clinical trials in infants of less than 1000 g birth weight have demonstrated that ICI is decreased 88% by antifungal prophylaxis with fluconazole compared to 54% by nystatin prophylaxis from retrospective studies. Fluconazole is more efficacious than nystatin prophylaxis in infants weighing less than 1000 g, is less expense, requires less frequent dosing (twice weekly intravenous [IV] dosing), and can be given when infants are not feeding. While antifungal prophylaxis is inexpensive, cost-effective, and easy to administer, yet has not been instituted universally despite A-1 evidence from single and multicenter studies demonstrating efficacy and safety. Debate is ongoing over whether empiric therapy or improved infection control practices are superior to prophylaxis, whether prophylaxis should be instituted only in neonatal intensive care units (NICUs) with a relatively high ICI rate, and whether fluconazole prophylaxis is safe or risks emergence of resistance. To date, azole resistance has not emerged with targeted treatment of high-risk infants for the duration of IV catheter use. Empiric therapy for suspected ICI and standardized therapy for candidemia, including central venous catheter removal, may decrease mortality; however, these approaches still risk neurodevelopmental impairment in ICI survivors. Infection control practices have not been subjected to prospective or randomized trials to demonstrate efficacy in reducing fungal infections. Evidence is presented in this article from clinical trials demonstrating efficacy and safety of antifungal prophylaxis in preventing ICI in preterm infants. The greatest impact of antifungal prophylaxis preventing ICI and decreasing Candida-related mortality and neurodevelopmental impairment would be achieved with a universal approach in all NICUs.

Ventilator-associated pneumonia (VAP) is one of the leading causes of preventable morbidity and mortality in neonatal intensive care units. This review examines the epidemiology and pathogenesis of VAP in neonates as well as the dilemmas faced by caregivers to diagnose and prevent VAP.

This article describes strategies to prevent 2 important healthcare associated infections in the neonatal intensive care unit: central line–associated bloodstream infections and catheter-associated urinary tract infections. Hand hygiene is discussed as the cornerstone for prevention of all healthcare associated infections. Specific recommendations for education and training of health care personnel who insert and maintain central venous catheters and urinary tract catheters are made and best practices for insertion and maintenance of these catheters are discussed. Throughout this article, the emphasis is on prevention of these high morbidity and mortality healthcare associated infections.

The clinical outcome of central nervous system infection is determined by the characteristics of the pathogen and the brain's response to the invading bacteria. How infection leads to brain injury remains unresolved. An impediment to progress is the complexity of pathophysiologic processes. Some of the mechanisms involved have been identified in experimental models, providing insights into the molecular basis of brain injury and regeneration, and hinting at targets for therapy. Adjuvant therapies have been proposed. Interventions that protect the brain are evaluated for their potential to preserve neuro-integrative functions in long-term survivors of bacterial meningitis. This article summarizes current studies evaluating pharmacologic interventions in experimental models of bacterial meningitis and discusses how the knowledge gathered could translate into more effective therapies.

Current strategies to prevent infection-related preterm birth and its associated neonatal morbidities have had limited success. Improved understanding of the pathogen-host interactions underlying altered colonization of the lower genital tract is necessary before significant progress can be made. The application of novel diagnostic techniques such as broad range PCR and proteomic analysis contribute to our knowledge of the diversity and abundance of microbial species invading the amniotic cavity as well as the resultant inflammatory response. Preterm infants delivered following intrauterine infection may respond differently to subsequent infectious challenges in the neonatal intensive care unit.

GOAL STATEMENT

The goal of *Clinics in Perinatology* is to keep practicing neonatologists and maternal-fetal medicine specialists up to date with current clinical practice in perinatology by providing timely articles reviewing the state of the art in patient care.

ACCREDITATION

The *Clinics in Perinatology* is planned and implemented in accordance with the Essential Areas and Policies of the Accreditation Council for Continuing Medical Education (ACCME) through the joint sponsorship of the University of Virginia School of Medicine and Elsevier. The University of Virginia School of Medicine is accredited by the ACCME to provide continuing medical education for physicians.

The University of Virginia School of Medicine designates this educational activity for a maximum of 15 *AMA PRA Category 1 Credits*™ for each issue, 60 credits per year. Physicians should only claim credit commensurate with the extent of their participation in the activity.

The American Medical Association has determined that physicians not licensed in the US who participate in this CME activity are eligible for a maximum of 15 *AMA PRA Category 1 Credits*™ for each issue, 60 credits per year.

Credit can be earned by reading the text material, taking the CME examination online at http://www.theclinics.com/home/cme, and completing the evaluation. After taking the test, you will be required to review any and all incorrect answers. Following completion of the test and evaluation, your credit will be awarded and you may print your certificate.

FACULTY DISCLOSURE/CONFLICT OF INTEREST

The University of Virginia School of Medicine, as an ACCME accredited provider, endorses and strives to comply with the Accreditation Council for Continuing Medical Education (ACCME) Standards of Commercial Support, Commonwealth of Virginia statutes, University of Virginia policies and procedures, and associated federal and private regulations and guidelines on the need for disclosure and monitoring of proprietary and financial interests that may affect the scientific integrity and balance of content delivered in continuing medical education activities under our auspices.

The University of Virginia School of Medicine requires that all CME activities accredited through this institution be developed independently and be scientifically rigorous, balanced and objective in the presentation/discussion of its content, theories and practices.

All authors/editors participating in an accredited CME activity are expected to disclose to the readers relevant financial relationships with commercial entities occurring within the past 12 months (such as grants or research support, employee, consultant, stock holder, member of speakers bureau, etc.). The University of Virginia School of Medicine will employ appropriate mechanisms to resolve potential conflicts of interest to maintain the standards of fair and balanced education to the reader. Questions about specific strategies can be directed to the Office of Continuing Medical Education, University of Virginia School of Medicine, Charlottesville, Virginia.

The faculty and staff of the University of Virginia Office of Continuing Medical Education have no financial affiliations to disclose.

The authors/editors listed below have identified no professional or financial affiliations for themselves or their spouse/partner:
Robert Boyle, MD (Test Author); Alison J. Carey, MD; Karen D. Fairchild, MD (Guest Editor); Philip L. Graham III, MD, MSc; Denis Grandgirard, PhD; Carla Holloway (Acquisitions Editor); David A. Kaufman, MD; Hugh S. Lam, MRCPCH; Sarah S. Long, MD; Pak C Ng, MD, FRCPCH; T. Michael O'Shea, MD; Sameer J. Patel, MD; Tara M. Randis, MD; Lisa Saiman, MD, MPH; and Michael P. Sherman, MD.

The authors/editors listed below identified the following professional or financial affiliations for themselves or their spouse/partner:
Jeffery S. Garland, MD, SM serves on the Advisory Committee/Board for Ethicon Inc.
Stephen L. Leib, MD serves on the Advisory Committee and is an industry funded research/investigator for Cubist Pharmaceutical and Novartis Pharmaceuticals.
Paolo Manzoni, MD serves on the Advisory Committee for Astellas.
Richard A. Polin, MD (Guest Editor) serves on the Advisory Committee for Discovery Laboratory.

Disclosure of Discussion of Non-FDA Approved Uses for Pharmaceutical Products and/or Medical Devices.

The University of Virginia School of Medicine, as an ACCME provider, requires that all faculty presenters identify and disclose any off-label uses for pharmaceutical and medical device products. The University of Virginia School of Medicine recommends that each physician fully review all the available data on new products or procedures prior to clinical use.

TO ENROLL

To enroll in the Clinics in Perinatology Continuing Medical Education program, call customer service at 1-800-654-2452 or visit us online at www.theclinics.com/home/cme. The CME program is available to subscribers for an additional fee of $196.00

RELATED INTEREST

Clinics in Perinatology, March 2008 (Volume 35, Issue 1)
Iatrogenic Disease
Marcus C. Hermansen, MD, *Guest Editor*
www.perinatology.theclinics.com

THE CLINICS ARE NOW AVAILABLE ONLINE!

Access your subscription at:
www.theclinics.com

Preface: Healthcare Associated Infections in the Neonatal Intensive Care Unit

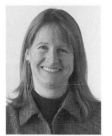 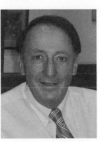

Karen D. Fairchild, MD   Richard A. Polin, MD
Guest Editors

This issue of *Clinics in Perinatology* focuses on healthcare associated infections (HAIs) in the neonatal intensive care unit (NICU). Although early-onset infections are often more dramatic in their presentation, HAIs are 50-100 times more common in neonates, increase length of stay, and add tens of millions of dollars to annual healthcare expenditures. For many years the assumption has been that most HAIs in the NICU are not preventable and cause minimal morbidity and mortality. In fact, the converse is true; most HAIs in neonates are preventable, and these infections (even those due to "low virulence organisms") are associated with increased mortality and morbidities, including neurodevelopmental impairment.

This issue of *Clinics in Perinatology* focuses on the epidemiology, diagnosis, treatment, and prevention of HAIs in the NICU. In the first article, Drs Carey and Long review the epidemiology and presentation of *Staphylococcus aureus* infections. Methicillin-susceptible and -resistant Staphylococci are becoming increasingly common pathogens in the NICU and well-baby nursery. That is particularly true for community-acquired staphylococci, which are often resistant to commonly used antibiotics. Eradication of carriage is difficult and attempts at passive protection using monoclonal antibodies have not proven efficacious.

The next article by Patel and Saiman focuses on a closely related issue: the development of antimicrobial-resistant pathogens. Resistant microorganisms (notably vancomycin-resistant enterococci, Methicillin-resistant *S aureus*, and extended spectrum beta-lactamase producing gram-negative bacteria) are becoming more prevalent in the NICU. Strategies to limit the development of resistant microorganisms include judicious use of antibiotics, development of an antibiotic stewardship program, surveillance for resistant bacteria, and infection control measures to limit the acquisition

Clin Perinatol 37 (2010) xi–xiii
doi:10.1016/j.clp.2010.06.006   perinatology.theclinics.com
0095-5108/10/$ – see front matter © 2010 Elsevier Inc. All rights reserved.

and spread of resistant microorganisms. A multidisciplinary approach that includes all of those interventions is likely to be most effective.

The article by Sherman discusses the importance bacterial translocation in pathogenesis of necrotizing enterocolitis (NEC) and neonatal sepsis. Because the gut appears to be a major pathway for infection and tissue injury in the neonate, there are a number of potential interventions to lessen the probability of sepsis or NEC. These include breast milk feeding, use of pre- and probiotics, and enhancing intestinal immunity. Recent clinical data strongly support lactoferrin for sepsis prevention in preterm infants and randomized clinical trials are in progress.

Fairchild and O'Shea and Ng and Lam discuss new ways to diagnose HAIs in the NICU. Fairchild and O'Shea review the rationale and efficacy of continuous monitoring of heart rate characteristics. There is increasing evidence that a systemic inflammatory response may alter heart rate patterns (by altering autonomic function) and provide a very early warning that sepsis is present. However, other disease processes (eg, cardiovascular disease, hypoxia, and brain injury) can also affect heart rate variability and the clinical utility of heart rate monitoring for predicting sepsis events will await the results of a large clinical trial nearing completion. The article by Ng and Lam discusses the role of biomarkers in the early diagnosis of sepsis. Although there is no ideal biomarker, the use of proteomics in combination with cytokine determinations may lead to development of automated systems for detection of sepsis before culture results are known. However, it is not clear at present if these biomarkers are superior to conventional diagnostic testing (acute phase reactants and neutrophil indices).

In the next article, Drs Kaufman and Manzoni review the data in support of fluconazole prophylaxis to prevent invasive fungal infections in extremely low birth weight infants. Although the data are compelling, it is not yet recommended as routine by national and international infectious disease organizations. Nonetheless, prophylaxis may make clinical and economic sense in NICUs with a relatively high incidence of infections caused by *Candida sp.*

The next two articles review strategies to prevent ventilator-associated pneumonia (VAP) (Garland) and catheter-associated bloodstream infections (Graham). VAP is a poorly described (and therefore underreported) entity in the NICU. It is difficult to diagnose VAP in a ventilated neonate because of the many noninfectious conditions that mimic VAP (eg, bronchopulmonary dysplasia). Furthermore, preventative strategies of benefit in the adult population have not been systematically tested in neonates. Catheter-related bloodstream infections represent the largest category of HAIs in the neonate. Fortunately, most of these infections are preventable by good hand hygiene practices and "infection control bundles" that focus on catheter insertion and maintenance techniques.

The Grandgirard and Leib article reviews the pathogenesis of neonatal meningitis and the pathophysiology of brain injury in affected infants. Meningitis occurs in 5%-10% of neonates with late-onset sepsis and is associated with an increased likelihood of a poor neurodevelopmental outcome. Although prevention of infections is still most important, there are a number of potential strategies to lessen brain injury in infants with central nervous system infections.

The final article by Randis reviews the relationship between antenatal infection and preterm birth. Although prematurity is a major risk factor for development of an HAI, intrauterine infections may alter the ability of the preterm infant to respond to an infectious challenge. Furthermore, the immune response to intrauterine infection may lead to long-term morbidities such as bronchopulmonary dysplasia and periventricular leukomalacia.

We dedicate this issue to our families for their support and incredible patience. We are also indebted to Carla Holloway at Elsevier for her editorial assistance and help with the organization of this *Clinics in Perinatology* issue.

Karen D. Fairchild, MD
Department of Pediatrics
Division of Neonatology
University of Virginia Hospital
Box 800386 Charlottesville
VA 22908, USA

Richard A. Polin, MD
Department of Pediatrics
Division of Neonatology
College of Physicians and Surgeons
Columbia University, New York, NY, USA

Morgan Stanley Children's Hospital of New York
3959 Broadway, CHC 115
New York, NY 10032, USA

E-mail addresses:
KDF2N@hscmail.mcc.virginia.edu (K.D. Fairchild)
rap32@columbia.edu (R.A. Polin)

Staphylococcus aureus: A Continuously Evolving and Formidable Pathogen in the Neonatal Intensive Care Unit

Alison J. Carey, MD[a],*, Sarah S. Long, MD[b]

KEYWORDS

• Staphylococcus aureus • MRSA • MSSA • Neonates

Staphylococcus aureus has long been a problem in the newborn period. As early as 1937, guidance for proper skin care of newborns was given to prevent staphylococcal infection.[1] The first description of a penicillin-resistant S aureus outbreak in the newborn nursery was in 1952,[2] when chlortetracycline (Aureomycin), the first of the tetracyclines, was used for the treatment of pustular dermatitis, conjunctivitis, and pneumonia. Around this time, a virulent strain of S aureus of the 52/52A/80/81 phage complex causing infections in neonates and their family contacts was first described.[3] In response to outbreaks of this virulent strain in nurseries, Shinefield and colleagues[4–7] investigated the method of artificial colonization, in which neonates were colonized purposefully with the less-virulent S aureus 502A strain, in attempts to compete with or prevent colonization of more virulent S aureus. Artificial colonization successfully controlled S aureus outbreaks in Ohio and Georgia.

Since the 1970s, methicillin-resistant S aureus (MRSA) has been a major pathogen in hospital-associated MRSA (HA-MRSA) infections[8] and was first described in the neonatal intensive care unit (NICU) in 1981.[9] However, in the 1990s, a global epidemic of community-associated MRSA (CA-MRSA) infections began to cause infections in

[a] Division of Neonatology, St Christopher's Hospital for Children, 3601 A Street, Philadelphia, PA 19134, USA
[b] Division of Infectious Diseases, St Christopher's Hospital for Children, 3601 A Street, Philadelphia, PA 19134, USA
* Corresponding author.
E-mail address: alison.carey@drexelmed.edu

Clin Perinatol 37 (2010) 535–546
doi:10.1016/j.clp.2010.05.002   **perinatology.theclinics.com**

people without traditional risk factors. At present, MRSA is responsible for almost 60% of skin and soft tissue S aureus infections in children's hospitals in United States,[10] and CA-MRSA causes up to 74% of skin and soft tissue S aureus infections in adults presenting to emergency departments, depending on the regional incidence of MRSA.[11] In highly endemic areas, such as Texas, nasal colonization rates have been reported as high as 20%.[12] Outbreaks of CA-MRSA have been associated with crowding, skin conditions, and skin-to-skin contact, such as in sports teams, schools, prison inmates,[13] men who have sex with men,[14] and personnel in military barracks.[15] In addition, there have been HA outbreaks among postpartum women[16] and infants in well-newborn nursery,[17] settings that are often overcrowded and under-staffed. There have been various reports of vaginal colonization with MRSA, with rates ranging from 0.5% to 10.4%.[18-20] These women could act as potential reservoirs of MRSA and transmit this pathogen to their infants at the time of delivery.

Recently, methicillin-susceptible S aureus (MSSA) seems to have acquired virulence factors from CA-MRSA, leading to a highly transmissible and virulent disease indistinguishable from that of CA-MRSA. This review focuses on the evolution of S aureus causing infections during the newborn period and the management of such infections in this new era of S aureus.

EPIDEMIOLOGY

The National Institute of Child Health and Human Development (NICHD) Neonatal Research Network maintains a prospective registry of early- and late-onset infections among very low-birth-weight (VLBW; ≤1500 g) infants. S aureus is a rare cause of early-onset sepsis in VLBW infants. In an evaluation of 5447 VLBW infants between 1998 and 2000, 84 patients had early-onset septicemia of which only 1 patient was infected with S aureus,[21] and this low incidence was confirmed in a more recent (2002-2003) data analysis as well.[22] In contrast, 7.8% of all first episodes of late-onset sepsis were due to S aureus.[23]

These reports did not distinguish MSSA and MRSA isolates. However, MSSA and MRSA are reported in neonatal data from the National Nosocomial Infections Surveillance System, 1995-2004.[24] MRSA accounted for 23% of HA S aureus infections; the incidence of MRSA infections increased by 308% during the study period and was similar across all birth-weight categories. In more recent years, 30% of S aureus infections in a level III NICU were caused by MRSA (**Fig. 1**).[25]

In recent years, disease caused by CA-MRSA in NICUs,[26,27] previously healthy neonates,[28] and children in the community[29,30] has been predominantly due to the USA300 clone. This strain is a major cause of skin and soft tissue infections (SSTIs) in both the community and health care setting. There are 20 genes unique to USA300 isolates, which distinguish this strain from HA-MRSA isolates typical of the 1980s and early 1990s. It is likely that USA300 contains additional virulence loci that are yet to be elucidated.[31]

RESISTANCE AND VIRULENCE FACTORS

The staphylococcal chromosome cassette (SCC) mecA has the genes responsible for antibiotic resistance, including mecA, which encodes for the penicillin-binding protein 2A (PBP 2A). PBP 2A has much lower affinity for β-lactam antibiotics when compared with natural binding proteins, thus interrupting the mechanism by which the β-lactam antibiotics block cell wall synthesis.[32]

Different SCC mec types are associated with the previous decade's classic HA-MRSA (SCC mecA I–III) and the current epidemic CA-MRSA (type SCC mecA IV–V).

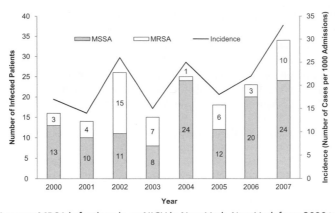

Fig. 1. MSSA versus MRSA infections in an NICU in New York, New York from 2000 to 2007. Infections caused by MSSA and MRSA are shown as the number of infected patients (left hand y-axis) and as the number of cases per 1000 patient admissions (right hand y-axis). The number of infected infants in each year is shown within the bars. (*From* Carey AJ, Duchon J, Della-Latta P, et al. The epidemiology of methicillin-susceptible and methicillin-resistant *Staphylococcus aureus* in a neonatal intensive care unit, 2000–2007. J Perinatol 2010;30(2):137; with permission.)

Classic HA-MRSA is characterized by a multidrug-resistant antibiogram pattern, because the SCC harbors multiple resistance determinants. In contrast, CA-MRSA is usually susceptible to some non–β-lactam antibiotics, such as trimethoprim-sulfamethoxazole, clindamycin, aminoglycosides, and quinolones.[33] Because of its large and cumbersome chromosomal cassette that encodes multidrug resistance, classic HA-MRSA suffered a fitness disadvantage (eg, metabolic requirements to maintain resistance genes, loss of transmissibility, and loss of colonization advantage) and remained confined to health care settings in which there was favorable selective pressure. Whereas, CA-MRSA has superadapted, with no fitness cost of resistance genes. In the last decade in NICUs, CA-MRSA has replaced HA-MRSA as a more common cause of infections.[27,34]

Superadapted CA-MRSA also has multiple transmissibility and virulence factors. Some strains express Panton-Valentine leukocidin (PVL) and staphylococcal enterotoxins, which have been implicated as potential virulence factors in SSTIs.[16] The *pvl* genes lead to the production of cytotoxins that form pores in cellular membranes causing tissue necrosis and cell lysis.[32] These toxins may explain the furunculosis and severe necrotizing pneumonia that are highly associated with CA *S aureus*.[35] In a study of national rates of MRSA colonization, only 8% of isolates were positive for PVL.[36] In contrast, 42% of CA-MRSA strains of SCC *mec* Type IV clones have PVL,[37] and up to 78% of the omnipresent USA300 MRSA clones carry PVL.[38]

The role of PVL in the pathogenesis of *S aureus* is controversial. An unintended point mutation in the *agr* P2 promoter of *S aureus* was shown to cause the phenotype of pneumonia attributed to PVL by earlier investigators.[39] PVL may not be the actual virulence factor, but may be hitchhiking with other genes, and is simply a marker for other virulence factors. Other investigators have proposed that the discrepancy of the role of PVL in virulence may be the result of differences in toxin expression between individual strains.[40] Changes in the production of PVL may be the result of changes in promoter sequences, regulators, or other factors that affect protein levels.

There is a genomic region unique to the USA300 MRSA strain (compared with other sequenced *S aureus* strains), which is most closely related to a *S epidermidis* genomic pathogenicity island named arginine catabolic mobile element (ACME).[41] ACME contains several genes including those associated with arginine deiminase metabolism. There is controversy regarding the primary roles of virulence factors in causing the disease. McCaskill and colleagues[35] found that only 2 of the 29 isolates from invasive USA300 MSSA infections carried ACME, and they concluded that it was unlikely that this was a significant contributing factor to the increase in incidence of invasive infections due to USA300 MSSA. Some investigators have speculated that a few USA300 strains may have lost their SCC *mec* elements, thereby becoming MSSA or alternatively, the ancestor of CA-MRSA USA300 was an MSSA clone that acquired its resistance before spreading in the community.[42]

A BLURRED BORDER BETWEEN MRSA AND MSSA

Following the rapid increase in the number of CA-MRSA cases almost a decade ago, CA-MSSA is increasingly associated with severe and invasive disease. In fact, invasive disease is more often associated with CA-MSSA than with CA-MRSA isolates.[43] The USA300 clone (with its characteristic pathogenicity island) is not only increasing as MRSA isolates but also as CA-MSSA isolates. In a study from Houston, 25% of MSSA isolates were USA300 clones and these isolates were associated with more severe clinical presentations, evidenced by higher markers of inflammation and more frequent diagnosis of osteomyelitis.[35]

Apart from the lack of the SCC *mec* that confers methicillin resistance, genetic differences between USA300 MRSA and USA300 MSSA strains have not been described to date. The clinical presentations of the 2 strains are similar in terms of higher prevalence of osteomyelitis, in complications such as deep vein thrombosis with septic embolization of the lungs, and in deep skin, soft tissue, and lung infections. Therefore, the border between MRSA and MSSA is blurred, and one infection cannot be clinically distinguished from the other, particularly with the ongoing increase in the number of USA300 MSSA isolates. In addition, reports in both adults and children hospitalized with CA-*S aureus* infection showed that epidemiologic factors did not distinguish patients with CA-MRSA from those with CA-MSSA infections.[44,45]

CLINICAL MANIFESTATIONS

SSTIs, including osteomyelitis, surgical wound infections and cellulitis, are common manifestations of *S aureus* infections in neonates.[46–48] Compared with classic MSSA and HA-MRSA, CA-MRSA is highly associated with skin and skin structure infection and abscesses in adults and children.[49] There may also be a difference in the invasiveness of *S aureus* infections, with MSSA predominating among children with invasive infections and CA-MRSA predominating among children with SSTIs.[42,50]

In this regard, the NICU population may be different. In an 8-year study (2000–2007) in a level III NICU, the numbers of bloodstream infections (BSIs) and SSTIs remained stable for both MSSA and MRSA despite a shift from HA-MRSA to CA-MRSA.[25] There may be increased susceptibility to the development of BSIs in neonates because of the high prevalence of the use of central venous catheters, neonate's thin dermal barrier, and relative inability to contain infection.

S aureus poses multiple risks: persistent BSI, endovascular infection, thrombosis, and metastatic foci, such as pyogenic arthritis, osteomyelitis, visceral abscesses, brain abscesses, and septic embolic pneumonia. Delayed removal of infected indwelling catheters is an independent risk factor for developing serious complications of *S aureus* BSI.[51] To ensure an optimal outcome for a *S aureus* BSI, it is critical to remove devices immediately, repeatedly and meticulously examine each infant for subtle clues of focal infection, drain abscesses, and document the rapidity of sterilization of the bloodstream (with daily blood cultures) to plan the appropriate duration of therapy (**Fig. 2**). Primary pneumonia or pneumonia complicating ventilator therapy may also occur and is frequently complicated by alveolar necrosis, pneumatocele formation, and pleural empyema.

WELL-NEWBORN NURSERY

Although the NICU population is at great risk of developing nosocomial infections,[33] *S aureus* is not relegated solely to hospital units with critically ill, immunocompromised patients. In fact, *S aureus* is a serious threat in the well-newborn nursery. Skin infections with CA-MRSA (USA300) among otherwise healthy full-term newborns occurring within 30 days of delivery (typically during the second week of life) have been reported in Illinois,[52] California,[52] and Texas.[28] All neonates had an initial pustular vesicular exanthem, usually in the groin or perineum. Of note, most affected neonates were boys who were born by cesarean delivery.

Possible reasons for these associations are the longer hospital stays for neonates born by cesarean delivery and the additional procedure of circumcision for boys. On direct observation of the circumcision practices at the Los Angeles hospital with an outbreak in 2003 to 2004,[52] it was noted that the sterile equipment was left open for an extended period, there were lapses in hand hygiene practices by those performing the circumcisions, and uncovered, multiple-dose vials of lidocaine were used.[53] In addition, multiple manipulations with bandaging afford repeated opportunities for transmission from health care workers (HCWs) and parents.

In areas of high prevalence of MRSA, such as Houston, there have been reports of previously healthy term and late-preterm infants presenting within the first 30 days of

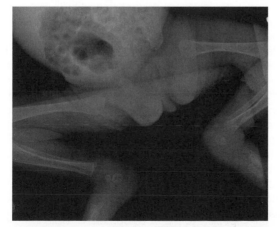

Fig. 2. Bone survey of the lower extremities in a 28-week gestation infant with persistently positive blood cultures with MSSA. Plain film of a 42-day-old, 28-week gestation girl baby who had a radiograph performed because of persistent MSSA bloodstream infection in the absence of a venous catheter. The mother noted crying when she elevated the hips to change the diaper. Examination revealed only mild swelling of the thigh compared with the other side and pain on movement of the hip. Demineralization of the proximal femur indicating osteomyelitis of at least 1-week duration can be observed. Joint aspiration and surgical debridement of the femur were performed, joint fluid culture was found to be negative, and a prolonged course of intravenous nafcillin was given.

delivery with SSTIs (some with invasive infection) due to *S aureus*. Most of these infections were caused by USA300 MRSA and were *pvl* positive.[28] Similarly, an outbreak of SSTIs (ie, pustulosis, cellulitis, and omphalitis) with USA400 occurred among infants discharged from a newborn nursery in Brooklyn, New York.[54]

TREATMENT

Vancomycin remains the first-line therapy for MRSA infections, and many NICUs with endemic MRSA use vancomycin as the empiric therapy for late-onset sepsis while awaiting culture results. However, the early development of vancomycin-insensitive *S aureus* has been observed in several studies reporting an increase in the minimum inhibitory concentrations (MICs).[55,56] Simply looking at categorical results of resistance or susceptibility, this relative decline in susceptibility, the so-called MIC creep, could not be detected. Increased MIC of 1 to 2 μg/mL, which is within the susceptible range, is a risk factor for vancomycin treatment failure in adults with invasive MRSA infections.[57] In addition, within a given clinical specimen, there can be heterogeneity among colonies, with a mixture of highly resistant and susceptible isolates. Therefore, infectious disease experts recommend a higher dose of vancomycin (eg, 15 mg/kg/ dose or more every 6 hours) in patients with serious infections to achieve consistent trough levels of 15 to 20 μg/mL,[58] particularly if the MIC is 1.0 μg/mL. For patients with isolates in which MIC of vancomycin is 2.0 μg/mL, another antibiotic should be substituted (eg, linezolid or clindamycin), depending on the susceptibility test results and site of clinical infection. Because linezolid and clindamycin are not usually bactericidal and clindamycin has no penetrance of the blood-brain barrier, care in coordination with a pediatric infectious disease expert is recommended.

Vancomycin is often combined with a second antibiotic, most often rifampin or gentamicin, for the treatment of serious MRSA infections. However, it has been shown that the addition of low-dose gentamicin for treating *S aureus* bacteremia and endocarditis is associated with increase in nephrotoxicity.[59] Patients most adversely affected by this treatment strategy have been those older than 65 years and with diabetes. Pediatric patients were not part of the study. Rifampin has many theoretically beneficial characteristics as an adjunctive agent to vancomycin (eg, activity in biofilms and ability to cross the blood-brain barrier); however, there are no clinical trial results that support the coadministration of rifampin.[60]

Although historically MSSA has been considered an endemic flora, MSSA infections can be as severe as MRSA infections in the pediatric population and may be more frequently associated with persistent BSIs. Until susceptibility results are known, some experts recommend concurrent empiric treatment with nafcillin and vancomycin for suspected *S aureus* infections in critically ill patients.[61] Nafcillin and oxacillin are more rapidly bactericidal than vancomycin for MSSA in vitro; for the treatment of MSSA bacteremic pneumonia in adults, clinical data suggest that nafcillin/oxacillin is superior to vancomycin.[62] Vancomycin attains poor concentrations in the pulmonary alveolar space. Furthermore, it has poor activity against organisms in the stationary growth phase[63] and in biofilms.[64]

PREVENTION

Risk factors for CA-MRSA versus HA-MRSA colonization in neonates hospitalized in NICUs include birth by vaginal delivery, endotracheal intubation, maternal substance abuse during pregnancy, and a higher gestational age and birth weight.[65]

It is difficult to determine the most effective measures for containment of MRSA, because during an outbreak, many measures are instituted concurrently. In 2006, a consensus statement was released from the Chicago Department of Public Health on management of outbreaks of MRSA in an NICU. Recommendations included alcohol-based rub for hand hygiene, regular neonatal surveillance cultures, and isolation and cohorting of MRSA-colonized babies.[66] Guidance emphasizes the use of molecular typing as an integral part of control to determine the ongoing transmission of a particular clone. Recommendations did not include attempting nasal decolonization with mupirocin; this intervention was left to the discretion of the primary clinical care team because the efficacy of this strategy is uncertain and mupirocin resistance exists. Routine chlorhexidine bathing of neonates in the absence of an outbreak setting has been relatively contraindicated in young infants, because of the potential risk of neurotoxicity from hexachlorophene.

Passive protection of neonates by using the monoclonal antibody tefibazumab, which binds to the surface-expressed adhesion protein clumping factor A, initially appeared promising[67] but has not proven to be efficacious. In addition, intravenous immunoglobulin derived from donors with high titers of antibody to surface adhesins of *Staphylococcus epidermidis* and *S aureus* has not been shown to prevent late-onset sepsis in VLBW infants.[68] It is controversial whether *S aureus* infection can be prevented by a vaccination approach. Carbohydrate surface molecules and polysaccharide-conjugate antigens may hold promise as vaccine candidates. However, vaccine strategy has multiple challenges: relevant antigens and immune responses, clinical endpoints, and universal versus targeted implementation.

Eradication of MRSA carriage may reduce the risk of subsequent MRSA infection in individuals and could decrease MRSA transmission by eliminating a reservoir for the organism. Attempts of decolonization have been unsuccessful because CA-MRSA has reservoirs at multiple body sites, not solely the anterior nares that were typical of CA-MSSA and HA-MRSA in the past. The likelihood of efficacy of topical nasal mupirocin alone to eradicate CA-MRSA is low and development of mupirocin resistance is substantial.[69,70] In a randomized study in adults, a regimen of intranasal mupirocin, daily showers with chlorhexidine gluconate 4%, along with rifampin and doxycycline orally was associated with a higher rate of decolonization compared with no treatment.[71] At 8 months postintervention and with sampling of multiple body sites, one-half of patients remained negative for MRSA colonization. Reduced risk of infection was not evaluated. Theoretically, reduction in time or density of MRSA colonization should decrease the transmissibility burden and potentially decrease the risk of infection. In one study, nasal mupirocin and chlorhexidine showers, although effective at decolonization, were not associated with decreased risk of infection.[72] These studies are generally performed in adult inpatient populations, and it is difficult to extrapolate the results to the NICU. Strategies that include intranasal mupirocin have been shown to control outbreaks of MRSA in NICUs,[73] but lack of sufficient data precludes recommendation for routine attempts to decolonize all MRSA carriers. Screening HCWs for colonization is not recommended, but educating all HCWs about hand hygiene as well as modes of *S aureus* transmission and excluding HCWs with active infection are critical.

A recent study reported the rates of MRSA colonization and infection in a single NICU over a 7-year-period (2000–2007) after implementation of routine weekly surveillance and contact isolation and patient cohorting.[74] There was an initial decrease in the incidence of MRSA colonization and infection to 0.15 cases per 1000 patient days from the peak of 1.79 cases per 1000 patient days in 2000, the beginning of the study period. However, by the end of the 7-year study period, the incidence had increased to 1.26 cases per 1000 patient days, and the antibiogram of colonized patients indicated a CA-MRSA type. Of note, the strategy implemented rested on screening and contact isolation and cohorting without topical decontaminating or decolonizing measures. This expensive ($1,500,000) and time-consuming surveillance program was not associated with sustained or complete control. The investigators speculated that the increase in MRSA colonization in the later part of the study period was due in part to increasing burden of MRSA colonization in the community, HCWs, and patients' family members. These are uncontrollable factors; nonetheless, halting transmission of MRSA and MSSA in NICUs continues to be the responsibility of HCWs.

SUMMARY AND FUTURE DIRECTIONS

S aureus is a particularly formidable pathogen in the neonate. The natural history of present MSSA/MRSA community-based epidemics suggests that control will be challenging and eradication impossible. Optimal management and prevention of S aureus infections in nurseries require well-designed, scientifically rigorous, prospective intervention, and outcome studies. These requirements are the opportunities to advance effective strategies and to direct research and development of novel approaches that might include vaccination, specific antibody or antimicrobial prophylaxis, or topical decontaminants.

REFERENCES

1. Sanford HN. Care of the skin of the newborn infant. J Pediatr 1937;11:68.
2. Feldman F, Annunziata D. Staphylococcus aureus infections in the newborn infant. J Pediatr 1952;41(4):399–402.
3. Colbeck JC. An extensive outbreak of staphylococcal infections in maternity units; the use of bacteriophage typing in investigation and control. Can Med Assoc J 1949;61(6):557–68.
4. Shinefield HR, Ribble JC, Boris M, et al. Bacterial interference: its effect on nursery-acquired infection with Staphylococcus aureus. I. Preliminary observations on artificial colonization of newborns. Am J Dis Child 1963;105:646–54.
5. Shinefield HR, Sutherland JM, Ribble JC, et al. Bacterial interference: its effect on nursery-acquired infection with Staphylococcus aureus. II. The Ohio epidemic. Am J Dis Child 1963;105:655–62.
6. Shinefield HR, Boris M, Ribble JC, et al. Bacterial interference: its effect on nursery-acquired infection with Staphylococcus aureus. III. The Georgia epidemic. Am J Dis Child 1963;105:663–73.
7. Shinefield HR, Ribble JC, Eichenwald HF, et al. Bacterial interference: its effect on nursery-acquired infection with Staphylococcus aureus. V. An analysis and interpretation. Am J Dis Child 1963;105:683–8.
8. Boyce JM. Increasing prevalence of methicillin-resistant Staphylococcus aureus in the United States. Infect Control Hosp Epidemiol 1990;11(12):639–42.
9. Weeks JL, Garcia-Prats JA, Baker CJ. Methicillin-resistant Staphylococcus aureus osteomyelitis in a neonate. JAMA 1981;245(16):1662–4.
10. Gerber JS, Coffin SE, Smathers SA, et al. Trends in the incidence of methicillin-resistant Staphylococcus aureus infection in children's hospitals in the United States. Clin Infect Dis 2009;49(1):65–71.
11. Moran GJ, Krishnadasan A, Gorwitz RJ, et al. Methicillin-resistant S. aureus infections among patients in the emergency department. N Engl J Med 2006;355(7):666–74.

12. Alfaro C, Mascher-Denen M, Fergie J, et al. Prevalence of methicillin-resistant *Staphylococcus aureus* nasal carriage in patients admitted to Driscoll Children's Hospital. Pediatr Infect Dis J 2006;25(5):459–61.
13. Lowy FD, Aiello AE, Bhat M, et al. *Staphylococcus aureus* colonization and infection in New York State prisons. J Infect Dis 2007;196(6):911–8.
14. Lee NE, Taylor MM, Bancroft E, et al. Risk factors for community-associated methicillin-resistant *Staphylococcus aureus* skin infections among HIV-positive men who have sex with men. Clin Infect Dis 2005;40(10):1529–34.
15. Zinderman CE, Conner B, Malakooti MA, et al. Community-acquired methicillin-resistant *Staphylococcus aureus* among military recruits. Emerg Infect Dis 2004;10(5):941–4.
16. Saiman L, O'Keefe M, Graham PL 3rd, et al. Hospital transmission of community-acquired methicillin-resistant *Staphylococcus aureus* among postpartum women. Clin Infect Dis 2003;37(10):1313–9.
17. James L, Gorwitz RJ, Jones RC, et al. Methicillin-resistant *Staphylococcus aureus* infections among healthy full-term newborns. Arch Dis Child Fetal Neonatal Ed 2008;93(1):F40–4.
18. Chen KT, Huard RC, Della-Latta P, et al. Prevalence of methicillin-sensitive and methicillin-resistant *Staphylococcus aureus* in pregnant women. Obstet Gynecol 2006;108(3 Pt 1):482–7.
19. Reusch M, Ghosh P, Ham C, et al. Prevalence of MRSA colonization in peripartum mothers and their newborn infants. Scand J Infect Dis 2008;40(8):667–71.
20. Creech CB, Litzner B, Talbot TR, et al. Frequency of detection of methicillin-resistant *Staphylococcus aureus* from rectovaginal swabs in pregnant women. Am J Infect Control 2010;38(1):72–4.
21. Stoll BJ, Hansen N, Fanaroff AA, et al. Changes in pathogens causing early-onset sepsis in very-low-birth-weight infants. N Engl J Med 2002;347(4):240–7.
22. Stoll BJ, Hansen NI, Higgins RD, et al. Very low birth weight preterm infants with early onset neonatal sepsis: the predominance of gram-negative infections continues in the National Institute of Child Health and Human Development Neonatal Research Network, 2002–2003. Pediatr Infect Dis J 2005; 24(7):635–9.
23. Stoll BJ, Hansen N, Fanaroff AA, et al. Late-onset sepsis in very low birth weight neonates: the experience of the NICHD Neonatal Research Network. Pediatrics 2002;110(2 Pt 1):285–91.
24. Lessa FC, Edwards JR, Fridkin SK, et al. Trends in incidence of late-onset methicillin-resistant *Staphylococcus aureus* infection in neonatal intensive care units: data from the National Nosocomial Infections Surveillance System, 1995–2004. Pediatr Infect Dis J 2009;28(7):577–81.
25. Carey AJ, Duchon J, Della-Latta P, et al. The epidemiology of methicillin-susceptible and methicillin-resistant *Staphylococcus aureus* in a neonatal intensive care unit, 2000–2007. J Perinatol 2010;30(2):135–9.
26. Healy CM, Hulten KG, Palazzi DL, et al. Emergence of new strains of methicillin-resistant *Staphylococcus aureus* in a neonatal intensive care unit. Clin Infect Dis 2004;39(10):1460–6.
27. McAdams RM, Ellis MW, Trevino S, et al. Spread of methicillin-resistant *Staphylococcus aureus* USA300 in a neonatal intensive care unit. Pediatr Int 2008;50(6): 810–5.
28. Fortunov RM, Hulten KG, Hammerman WA, et al. Community-acquired *Staphylococcus aureus* infections in term and near-term previously healthy neonates. Pediatrics 2006;118(3):874–81.

29. Chavez-Bueno S, Bozdogan B, Katz K, et al. Inducible clindamycin resistance and molecular epidemiologic trends of pediatric community-acquired methicillin-resistant *Staphylococcus aureus* in Dallas, Texas. Antimicrob Agents Chemother 2005;49(6):2283–8.

30. Buckingham SC, McDougal LK, Cathey LD, et al. Emergence of community-associated methicillin-resistant *Staphylococcus aureus* at a Memphis, Tennessee Children's Hospital. Pediatr Infect Dis J 2004;23(7):619–24.

31. Tenover FC, McDougal LK, Goering RV, et al. Characterization of a strain of community-associated methicillin-resistant *Staphylococcus aureus* widely disseminated in the United States. J Clin Microbiol 2006;44(1):108–18.

32. Diederen BM, Kluytmans JA. The emergence of infections with community-associated methicillin resistant *Staphylococcus aureus*. J Infect 2006;52(3): 157–68.

33. Carey AJ, Saiman L, Polin RA. Hospital-acquired infections in the NICU: epidemiology for the new millennium. Clin Perinatol 2008;35(1):223–49, x.

34. Carey AJ, Della-Latta P, Huard R, et al. Changes in the molecular epidemiological characteristics of methicillin-resistant *Staphylococcus aureus* in a neonatal intensive care unit. Infect Control Hosp Epidemiol 2010;31(6):613–9.

35. McCaskill ML, Mason EO Jr, Kaplan SL, et al. Increase of the USA300 clone among community-acquired methicillin-susceptible *Staphylococcus aureus* causing invasive infections. Pediatr Infect Dis J 2007;26(12):1122–7.

36. Graham PL 3rd, Lin SX, Larson EL. A U.S. population-based survey of *Staphylococcus aureus* colonization. Ann Intern Med 2006;144(5):318–25.

37. Davis SL, Rybak MJ, Amjad M, et al. Characteristics of patients with healthcare-associated infection due to SCCmec type IV methicillin-resistant *Staphylococcus aureus*. Infect Control Hosp Epidemiol 2006;27(10):1025–31.

38. Tsuji BT, Rybak MJ, Cheung CM, et al. Community- and health care-associated methicillin-resistant *Staphylococcus aureus*: a comparison of molecular epidemiology and antimicrobial activities of various agents. Diagn Microbiol Infect Dis 2007;58(1):41–7.

39. Villaruz AE, Bubeck Wardenburg J, Khan BA, et al. A point mutation in the agr locus rather than expression of the Panton-Valentine leukocidin caused previously reported phenotypes in *Staphylococcus aureus* pneumonia and gene regulation. J Infect Dis 2009;200(5):724–34.

40. Varshney AK, Martinez LR, Hamilton SM, et al. Augmented production of Panton-Valentine leukocidin toxin in methicillin-resistant and methicillin-susceptible *Staphylococcus aureus* is associated with worse outcome in a murine skin infection model. J Infect Dis 2010;201(1):92–6.

41. Diep BA, Gill SR, Chang RF, et al. Complete genome sequence of USA300, an epidemic clone of community-acquired methicillin-resistant *Staphylococcus aureus*. Lancet 2006;367(9512):731–9.

42. Mongkolrattanothai K, Aldag JC, Mankin P, et al. Epidemiology of community-onset *Staphylococcus aureus* infections in pediatric patients: an experience at a Children's Hospital in central Illinois. BMC Infect Dis 2009;9:112.

43. Kaplan SL, Hulten KG, Gonzalez BE, et al. Three-year surveillance of community-acquired *Staphylococcus aureus* infections in children. Clin Infect Dis 2005; 40(12):1785–91.

44. Faden H, Rose R, Lesse A, et al. Clinical and molecular characteristics of staphylococcal skin abscesses in children. J Pediatr 2007;151(6):700–3.

45. Miller LG, Perdreau-Remington F, Bayer AS, et al. Clinical and epidemiologic characteristics cannot distinguish community-associated methicillin-resistant

Staphylococcus aureus infection from methicillin-susceptible *S. aureus* infection: a prospective investigation. Clin Infect Dis 2007;44(4):471–82.

46. Davenport M, Doig CM. Wound infection in pediatric surgery: a study in 1,094 neonates. J Pediatr Surg 1993;28(1):26–30.

47. Korakaki E, Aligizakis A, Manoura A, et al. Methicillin-resistant *Staphylococcus aureus* osteomyelitis and septic arthritis in neonates: diagnosis and management. Jpn J Infect Dis 2007;60(2–3):129–31.

48. Friedland IR, du Plessis J, Cilliers A. Cardiac complications in children with *Staphylococcus aureus* bacteremia. J Pediatr 1995;127(5):746–8.

49. Jahamy H, Ganga R, Al Raiy B, et al. *Staphylococcus aureus* skin/soft-tissue infections: the impact of SCCmec type and Panton-Valentine leukocidin. Scand J Infect Dis 2008;40(8):601–6.

50. Sdougkos G, Chini V, Papanastasiou DA, et al. Community-associated *Staphylococcus aureus* infections and nasal carriage among children: molecular microbial data and clinical characteristics. Clin Microbiol Infect 2008;14(11):995–1001.

51. Fowler VG Jr, Justice A, Moore C, et al. Risk factors for hematogenous complications of intravascular catheter-associated *Staphylococcus aureus* bacteremia. Clin Infect Dis 2005;40(5):695–703.

52. Centers for Disease Control and Prevention (CDC). Community-associated methicillin-resistant *Staphylococcus aureus* infection among healthy newborns–Chicago and Los Angeles County, 2004. MMWR Morb Mortal Wkly Rep 2006; 55(12):329–32.

53. Nguyen DM, Bancroft E, Mascola L, et al. Risk factors for neonatal methicillin-resistant *Staphylococcus aureus* infection in a well-infant nursery. Infect Control Hosp Epidemiol 2007;28(4):406–11.

54. Bratu S, Eramo A, Kopec R, et al. Community-associated methicillin-resistant *Staphylococcus aureus* in hospital nursery and maternity units. Emerg Infect Dis 2005;11(6):808–13.

55. Steinkraus G, White R, Friedrich L. Vancomycin MIC creep in non-vancomycin-intermediate *Staphylococcus aureus* (VISA), vancomycin-susceptible clinical methicillin-resistant *S. aureus* (MRSA) blood isolates from 2001–05. J Antimicrob Chemother 2007;60(4):788–94.

56. Howden BP, Johnson PD, Charles PG, et al. Failure of vancomycin for treatment of methicillin-resistant *Staphylococcus aureus* infections. Clin Infect Dis 2004; 39(10):1544 [author reply: 1544–5].

57. Soriano A, Marco F, Martinez JA, et al. Influence of vancomycin minimum inhibitory concentration on the treatment of methicillin-resistant *Staphylococcus aureus* bacteremia. Clin Infect Dis 2008;46(2):193–200.

58. Frymoyer A, Hersh AL, Benet LZ, et al. Current recommended dosing of vancomycin for children with invasive methicillin-resistant *Staphylococcus aureus* infections is inadequate. Pediatr Infect Dis J 2009;28(5):398–402.

59. Cosgrove SE, Vigliani GA, Fowler VG Jr, et al. Initial low-dose gentamicin for *Staphylococcus aureus* bacteremia and endocarditis is nephrotoxic. Clin Infect Dis 2009;48(6):713–21.

60. Deresinski S. Vancomycin in combination with other antibiotics for the treatment of serious methicillin-resistant *Staphylococcus aureus* infections. Clin Infect Dis 2009;49(7):1072–9.

61. Kaplan SL. Community-acquired methicillin-resistant *Staphylococcus aureus* infections in children. Semin Pediatr Infect Dis 2006;17(3):113–9.

62. Gonzalez C, Rubio M, Romero-Vivas J, et al. Bacteremic pneumonia due to *Staphylococcus aureus*: a comparison of disease caused by

methicillin-resistant and methicillin-susceptible organisms. Clin Infect Dis 1999; 29(5):1171–7.

63. Lamp KC, Rybak MJ, Bailey EM, et al. In vitro pharmacodynamic effects of concentration, pH, and growth phase on serum bactericidal activities of daptomycin and vancomycin. Antimicrob Agents Chemother 1992;36(12):2709–14.

64. Rose WE, Poppens PT. Impact of biofilm on the in vitro activity of vancomycin alone and in combination with tigecycline and rifampicin against *Staphylococcus aureus*. J Antimicrob Chemother 2009;63(3):485–8.

65. Seybold U, Halvosa JS, White N, et al. Emergence of and risk factors for methicillin-resistant *Staphylococcus aureus* of community origin in intensive care nurseries. Pediatrics 2008;122(5):1039–46.

66. Gerber SI, Jones RC, Scott MV, et al. Management of outbreaks of methicillin-resistant *Staphylococcus aureus* infection in the neonatal intensive care unit: a consensus statement. Infect Control Hosp Epidemiol 2006;27(2):139–45.

67. Weems JJ Jr, Steinberg JP, Filler S, et al. Phase II, randomized, double-blind, multicenter study comparing the safety and pharmacokinetics of tefibazumab to placebo for treatment of *Staphylococcus aureus* bacteremia. Antimicrob Agents Chemother 2006;50(8):2751–5.

68. DeJonge M, Burchfield D, Bloom B, et al. Clinical trial of safety and efficacy of INH-A21 for the prevention of nosocomial staphylococcal bloodstream infection in premature infants. J Pediatr 2007;151(3):260–5, 265.e1.

69. Miller MA, Dascal A, Portnoy J, et al. Development of mupirocin resistance among methicillin-resistant *Staphylococcus aureus* after widespread use of nasal mupirocin ointment. Infect Control Hosp Epidemiol 1996;17(12):811–3.

70. Simor AE, Stuart TL, Louie L, et al. Mupirocin-resistant, methicillin-resistant *Staphylococcus aureus* strains in Canadian hospitals. Antimicrob Agents Chemother 2007;51(11):3880–6.

71. Simor AE, Phillips E, McGeer A, et al. Randomized controlled trial of chlorhexidine gluconate for washing, intranasal mupirocin, and rifampin and doxycycline versus no treatment for the eradication of methicillin-resistant *Staphylococcus aureus* colonization. Clin Infect Dis 2007;44(2):178–85.

72. Robicsek A, Beaumont JL, Thomson RB Jr, et al. Topical therapy for methicillin-resistant *Staphylococcus aureus* colonization: impact on infection risk. Infect Control Hosp Epidemiol 2009;30(7):623–32.

73. Hitomi S, Kubota M, Mori N, et al. Control of a methicillin-resistant *Staphylococcus aureus* outbreak in a neonatal intensive care unit by unselective use of nasal mupirocin ointment. J Hosp Infect 2000;46(2):123–9.

74. Gregory ML, Eichenwald EC, Puopolo KM. Seven-year experience with a surveillance program to reduce methicillin-resistant *Staphylococcus aureus* colonization in a neonatal intensive care unit. Pediatrics 2009;123(5):e790–6.

Antibiotic Resistance in Neonatal Intensive Care Unit Pathogens: Mechanisms, Clinical Impact, and Prevention Including Antibiotic Stewardship

Sameer J. Patel, MD[a], Lisa Saiman, MD, MPH[b,c,*]

KEYWORDS

• Antibiotic resistance • Neonatal intensive care unit • Prevention
• Antibiotic stewardship • Infection control

Antibiotic resistance is a public health crisis. The Institute of Medicine[1] has listed control and reduction of infections caused by antibiotic-resistant pathogens in acute care settings as one of the most important issues facing the medical community. The prevalence of antimicrobial-resistant (AMR) pathogens is higher in other intensive care unit (ICU) populations than in the neonatal ICU (NICU), but the experience in other populations is useful and can serve to warn NICU providers of the potential future threat. Thus, it is critical to understand the implications of the epidemiology of resistance to craft strategies to reduce AMR in the NICU population.

EPIDEMIOLOGY OF AMR ORGANISMS IN THE NICU

The epidemiology of pathogens causing hospital-acquired infections in the NICU population is well described, although it should be noted that most of the literature

[a] Department of Pediatrics, Columbia University, 622 West 168th Street, PH4W-475, New York, NY 10032, USA
[b] Department of Pediatrics, Columbia University, 622 West 168th Street, PH4W-470, New York, NY 10032, USA
[c] Department of Infection Prevention and Control, Morgan Stanley Children's Hospital of NewYork-Presbyterian, 177 Fort Washington, Milstein 7 Central, New York, NY 10032, USA
* Corresponding author. Department of Pediatrics, Columbia University, 622 West 168th Street, PH4W-470, New York, NY 10032.
E-mail address: Ls5@columbia.edu

Clin Perinatol 37 (2010) 547–563
doi:10.1016/j.clp.2010.06.004
0095-5108/10/$ – see front matter © 2010 Elsevier Inc. All rights reserved.

has focused on late-onset sepsis. Gram-positive pathogens are more common causes of infections than gram-negative pathogens and yeast.[2,3] Staphylococcal species, most notably *Staphylococcus epidermidis* and *Staphylococcus aureus*, cause approximately 60% to 70% of infections. *S epidermidis* is the most common gram-positive pathogen, although many clinical microbiology laboratories do not speciate coagulase-negative staphylococci; thus, the epidemiologic picture for other coagulase-negative staphylococci is incomplete. Gram-negative bacilli (GNB) cause approximately 15% to 20% of infections, most notably late-onset sepsis and hospital-acquired pneumonia, including ventilator-associated pneumonia. *Candida* spp cause approximately 10% of hospital-acquired infections in the NICU, most often candidemia and catheter-associated blood stream infections.

To date, most of the literature pertaining to AMR pathogens in the NICU reflects single-center reports rather than multicenter studies and thus may be skewed toward outbreaks rather than endemic infections.[4–6] Infants hospitalized in NICUs are at risk of developing colonization and infections caused by antibiotic-resistant organisms (AROs). Colonization with resistant organisms has implications for the colonized infant who can progress to infection and for other hospitalized infants because colonized infants may serve as a reservoir for AROs.[7]

Most hospital-acquired coagulase-negative staphylococci are resistant to oxacillin because of the *mecA* gene as described later. In addition, hospital-acquired coagulase-negative staphylococci are multidrug resistant, for example, resistant to gentamicin, rifampin, erythromycin, and clindamycin.[8] Thus, treatment options for synergy are limited for this pathogen. *Staphylococcus warneri* with higher minimal inhibitory concentrations (MICs) to vancomycin have been described, resulting in the concern for "MIC creep."[9] This concern seems well founded given the frequent use of empiric vancomycin in this population as well as selective pressure resulting from subtherapeutic concentrations of vancomycin at mucosal surfaces and sequestered sites, for example, biofilms within central venous catheters.

Methicillin-resistant *S aureus* (MRSA) is a critically important pathogen in the NICU population and has been associated with endemic and epidemic infections. In addition, the epidemiology of MRSA is changing from being exclusively a hospital-acquired pathogen to a pathogen with widespread distribution in the community capable of causing infection in otherwise healthy individuals. Similarly, the dominant MRSA clones in the NICU have been changing from hospital-associated (HA) to community-associated (CA) clones.[6] Reservoirs for MRSA include colonized infants in the NICU, staff members, the inanimate environment, and family members, including vertical transmission resulting from maternal anovaginal colonization in pregnancy.[10] Although hospital-acquired strains of MRSA in other patient populations are often multidrug resistant, strains in the NICU tend to be more susceptible; however, it is likely that this susceptibility varies according to local epidemiology and the dominant clone and the type of staphylococcal chromosomal cassette (SCC) present as described in the following sections. CA strains often harbor the virulence factor Panton-Valentine leukocidin and have been found to divide more rapidly than HA clones. USA300 is now the most common CA MRSA clone in the world and has been detected in NICUs.

In the NICU, enterococci are less-frequent pathogens than staphylococcal species. Nevertheless, ampicillin-resistant, and more recently, vancomycin-resistant enterococci have been described in the NICU.[11] Neither vancomycin-intermediate nor vancomycin-resistant coagulase-negative staphylococci or *S aureus* has been described in the NICU population.

GNB are becoming increasingly antibiotic resistant in health care settings and may be occasionally panresistant, that is, resistant to all conventional antibiotics. Although panresistant pathogens have been rare in the NICU, the increasing threat of multidrug-resistant GNB serves as a warning for close monitoring, infection control, and antibiotic stewardship, as described in later sections. In the NICU, the most common resistance patterns noted to date have been resistance to piperacillin-tazobactam, ceftazidime, and/or gentamicin.[12,13] More worrisome has been the emergence of extended-spectrum β-lactamase (ESBL)-producing pathogens that lead to resistance to third-generation cephalosporins, including cefotaxime, ceftriaxone, and ceftazidime, as well as the monobactam aztreonam.[14] *Klebsiella pneumonia* and *Escherichia coli* are most likely to acquire ESBLs, but these enzymes are also noted in other species.[15] Even more ominous, although not yet prevalent in pediatric populations, are the *K pneumoniae* carbapenemases (KPCs) that hydrolyze carbapenem agents, such as imipenem and meropenem, which are the treatment of choice for ESBL-producing pathogens.[16] Some GNB have become resistant to all first-line antibiotics and are only susceptible to polymyxin B and/or tigecycline, a tetracycline derivative. Quinolone resistance and tetracycline resistance are rare among pathogens isolated from patients in the NICU, presumably because these agents are rarely used in the NICU population.[6]

With the advent of fluconazole prophylaxis, aimed at preventing candidemia in very low–birth-weight (VLBW) or extremely low–birth-weight infants,[17,18] there has been concern about the emergence of resistance to fluconazole or the emergence of non-albicans or nonparapsilosis *Candida* spp such as has been observed in other populations.[19] During relatively short-term clinical trials (6–12 months), fluconazole resistance has not been detected in either infecting or colonizing flora.[17] However, more prolonged follow-up is likely needed to estimate the risk.

MECHANISMS OF ACTION AND MECHANISM OF RESISTANCE
Overview

An understanding of the mechanisms of resistance is predicated on an understanding of the mechanisms of action of antimicrobial agents. Briefly, antibacterial agents can bind to bacterial cell targets and prevent transcription (DNA to RNA) and translation (RNA to protein) or interfere with cell wall synthesis as described in **Table 1**. Antifungal agents have somewhat different mechanisms of action; amphotericin binds to ergosterol in fungal membranes causing leakage of fungal cell contents.[20] The azoles, including fluconazole, inhibit enzymes involved in ergosterol synthesis. The echiniocandins, which are not used frequently in the NICU, interfere with cell wall synthesis by binding to the protein complex that synthesizes cell wall 1,3-β-glucan polysaccharides.

Mechanisms of resistance for bacteria and yeast are characterized by 3 major mechanisms (see **Table 1**): (1) acquisition of an enzyme that alters the structure of an antibiotic, thereby rendering the agent unable to bind to the target of action; (2) mutations in the bacterial target site that prevent antibiotic binding (eg, mutations in penicillin-binding proteins [PBPs], DNA gyrase, or the proteins involved in ergosterol biosynthesis); or (3) changes in uptake via multidrug efflux pumps, which remove antibiotics from the microorganism, or changes in porins, which prevent antibiotic entry into bacterial cells.

Microorganisms continually mutate; some mutations are silent, some are lethal, and some confer a selective advantage. Bacteria are also avid at acquiring new DNA from other bacteria, which may be located on plasmids that often carry multiple-resistance

Table 1
Commonly used antibiotics in the NICU and mechanisms of action and resistance

Major Classes of Antibacterial Agents	Examples of Specific Antimicrobial Agents	Mechanisms of Action	Mechanisms of Resistance
β-Lactam agents Penicillins	Penicillin/ampicillin/oxacillin	Interfere with bacterial cell wall synthesis by binding to transpeptidase active site of PBP	Acquisition of β-lactamases, which hydrolyze β-actam ring Mutations in PBP Loss of porins
Cephalosporins	First generation: cefazolin Second generation: cefoxitin Third generation: cefotaxime		
Carbapenems	Meropenem/imipenem		
Aminoglycosides	Gentamicin Tobramycin Amikacin	Interfere with protein synthesis by binding to 30S ribosomal subunit	Acquisition of aminoglycoside-modifying enzymes that alter drug side chains
Glycopeptides	Vancomycin	Interfere with bacterial cell wall synthesis by binding to C-terminal D-alanine–D-alanine	Mutation in terminal component of cell wall, leading to alteration from D-alanine–D-alanine to D-alanine–D-lactate

Abbreviation: PBP, penicillin-binding protein.

genes. Thus, mutations that result in antibiotic resistance are highly desirable from the microorganism's perspective.

The Impact of β-Lactamases

As shown in **Table 1**, β-lactam agents bind to PBPs, which help to construct new cell wall for dividing bacteria. Gram-negative and gram-positive bacteria can possess different types of PBPs in varying concentrations. Furthermore, agents differ in their affinity for a given PBP. For example, the major target of broad-spectrum carbapenem agents (with activity against both gram-negative and gram-positive pathogens) is PBP2.

All β-lactam agents (penicillins, cephalosporins, monobactams, and carbapenems) possess β-lactam rings. β-Lactamases hydrolyze the ring and alter the configuration of the antibiotic such that the antibiotic can no longer bind to the PBP. There are dozens of β-lactamases with different affinities for different antibiotics. For example, some enzymes preferentially hydrolyze penicillins, whereas others hydrolyze cephalosporins. Such enzymes are inhibited by the β-lactamase inhibitors sulbactam (combined with ampicillin) or tazobactam (combined with ticarcillin). As mentioned earlier, β-lactamases can hydrolyze third-generation cephalosporins, that is, the ESBLs, whereas others can hydrolyze carbapenems, that is, the KPCs. Some β-lactamases are carried on plasmids, which can facilitate transfer to other bacterial cells, whereas others are located within the chromosome. The nomenclature and spectrum of activity of β-lactamases are complex and have been recently reviewed.[21]

MRSA: CA Versus HA Strains

Resistance to oxacillin in *S aureus* and coagulase-negative staphylococci is because of acquisition of *mecA*, which is contained on the SCC as recently reviewed.[22] *mecA* does not code for a β-lactamase but rather for a PBP2 with low affinity for β-lactam agents.[23] Differences in the genetic composition of SCC are the basis for the different phenotypes of CA and HA MRSA (**Table 2**). However, the phenotypic distinction between CA and HA strains is gradually blurring because CA strains are becoming increasingly resistant.

Resistance to Vancomycin

Thus far, resistance to vancomycin (initially described during the 1990s) has largely been limited to *Enterococcus faecium*, although there are reports of vancomycin resistance in *Enterococcus faecalis*. *E faecalis* is more likely to be susceptible to ampicillin as well. Resistance to vancomycin occurs by 2 mechanisms: *vanA* or *vanB*; these gene clusters alter the vancomycin target from D-alanine–D-alanine to D-alanine–D-lactate.[24]

Resistance to vancomycin has also been reported in *S aureus*, although the *vanA* and *vanB* gene clusters noted in enterococci have, thus far, rarely been noted in staphylococci. Instead, intermediate vancomycin resistance has been well described, which is mediated by alterations in cell wall structure, including a thickened capsule and thickened wall, which presumably limit the access of vancomycin to its D-alanine–D-alanine target.[23] Another phenotype of vancomycin resistance is heteroresistance whereby in vitro susceptibility testing of a single strain reveals both susceptible bacterial cells (MIC ≤ 2 μg/mL) and intermediately resistant cells (MIC ≤ 4–8 μg/mL). Heteroresistance can be difficult to detect in the laboratory but may have clinical implications as described later.

Table 2
Comparison of CA MRSA versus HA MRSA

Characteristic	CA MRSA	HA MRSA	Comment
mecA	Present	Present	Encodes for PBP2a
SCCmecA	IV and V Relatively small, about 20 kb	I, II, III Relatively large, more than 30 kb Carry additional resistance genes	USA300 is the most common CA clone
Resistance pattern	Resistant to oxacillin and other β-lactam agents	Resistant to Oxacillin and other β-lactam agents Rifampin Gentamicin Erythromycin Tetracycline Clindamycin Trimethoprim sulfamethoxazole	CA strains are increasingly resistant

CLINICAL IMPACT OF AMR PATHOGENS

The mortality and morbidity of AROs may be related to increased virulence, delay in appropriate therapy, and fewer treatment options. Furthermore, antimicrobials required to treat AROs may be less effective, more expensive, or more toxic than conventional therapy. Resistance may be difficult to detect, can cause increased costs and length of stay, and may lead to a vicious cycle of antibiotic overuse, as broader empiric choices are then required. However, attributable mortality to AMR is difficult to measure because critically ill neonates with infections caused by AROs often have comorbid conditions.

Numerous outbreaks of MRSA have been reported in the NICU.[25,26] MRSA infections typically manifest as skin, eye, and blood stream infections, although other invasive infections can occur.[9,27–29] In a 7-year retrospective study of 172 S aureus infections occurring in a tertiary care NICU, methicillin-susceptible S aureus (MSSA) caused 123 (72%) infections and MRSA caused 49 (28%) infections, most commonly, bacteremia and skin and soft tissue infections.[27] The types of infections caused by MSSA and MRSA were similar. Although infants with MRSA were younger at presentation, crude mortality was not different. Infected infants exhibited a bimodal weight distribution (potentially because of the large number of full-term infants with congenital anomalies cared for at this NICU); 53% of S aureus infections occurred in extremely low–birth-weight infants who were less than 1000 g, and 27% occurred among term infants with birth weights more than 2500 g, most of whom had undergone surgical procedures. Similarly, Cohen-Wolkowiez and colleagues[30] described a comparable crude mortality rate between infants with MRSA and MSSA blood stream infections, although duration of bacteremia was longer in infants infected with MRSA (4.5 days vs 1 day, respectively). Management of MRSA in NICUs is further complicated by the complexity of using vancomycin because this agent requires dose adjustment for postconception age, renal insufficiency, receipt of extracorporeal membrane oxygenation, and body site of infection.[31] Failure to adjust dosing may lead to low troughs, which may lead to treatment failures, particularly for sequestered sites, such as the lung or the central nervous system.

As described earlier, CA MRSA strains have emerged as a significant cause of infections in the NICU. CA MRSA strains, like HA MRSA strains, typically cause skin and soft tissue infections, although bacteremia, pneumonia, and meningitis can also occur.[32–34] Kuint and colleagues[35] demonstrated that although infants with CA MRSA bacteremia were more premature than infants with HA MRSA or MSSA bacteremia, mortality rates did not differ. CA MRSA infections have caused outbreaks in maternity wards and well-baby nurseries, including skin infections among otherwise healthy full-term newborns and mastitis and postpartum infections among mothers.[10,36]

Neonatal bacteremia is most frequently caused by coagulase-negative staphylococcal strains with high rates of *mecA* gene carriage. These strains have been found to be harbored by neonates and staff, suggesting cross-transmission of resistant strains.[37–39] *S warneri* has been demonstrated to be an important pathogen in the NICU, with decreased vancomycin susceptibility.[40] This observation is particularly of concern because such strains can be shared between neonates and nurses' hands.[9] In one case report, a neonate with 3 weeks of persistently positive blood cultures for *Staphylococcus capitis* was found to be infected with a strain that was heteroresistant to vancomycin.[41] As conventional antibiotic testing may indicate susceptibility, treatment failure (despite removal of central venous catheters) may be because of heteroresistance. Perhaps more concerning, Villari and colleagues[42] described 81 *S epidermidis* isolates, including 27 from blood stream infections, most of which demonstrated heterogeneous vancomycin susceptibility, although the clinical implications of this was uncertain.

Manifestations of vancomycin-resistant *Enterococcus* (VRE) infection have included bacteremia, meningitis, and endocarditis.[43–47] McNeeley and colleagues[48] reported a significantly greater mean age of onset for VRE bacteremia than for infections caused by vancomycin-susceptible *Enterococci* (101 vs 34 days, respectively). The clinical presentations of VRE versus susceptible strains were indistinguishable, but infants with VRE bacteremia had significantly higher crude mortality (0 of 6 vs 72 of 94), potentially due to comorbid conditions. Furthermore, conclusions are limited by the small sample size. Epidemiologic investigations following VRE infections have consistently demonstrated a higher ratio of colonized infants to infected infants.[49,50] Thus, a single positive clinical infection may represent a hidden reservoir of colonization.[50] Antibiotic options in VRE infections are limited to bacteriostatic agents, usually linezolid, which have not been evaluated in large studies in neonatal populations.[43,44,50]

Increasing AMR among GNB is of particular concern because many institutions have reported an increased proportion of blood stream infections caused by GNB.[3,51,52] Numerous publications from NICUs in the developed and developing world have described outbreaks of antibiotic-resistant gram-negative pathogens with well-characterized mechanisms of resistance. ESBL-producing *Enterobacter hormaechei* caused 5 episodes of sepsis in neonates in California during 6 months,[53] and ESBL-producing GNB have caused early-onset sepsis, suggesting potential maternal colonization in the community.[54] Jeena and colleagues[55] described an outbreak of multidrug-resistant *Acinetobacter anitratus* in a pediatric and neonatal ICU, causing 23 infections, primarily postoperative infections and pneumonia, with a 57% mortality rate. Birth weight less than 1000 g and receipt of prolonged antibiotic therapy (>21 days) have been associated with increased risk of infections caused by antibiotic-resistant GNB.[56] In developing countries, where GNB cause a larger proportion of neonatal sepsis than in developed countries, the burden of resistance is even greater. In a large 10-year study of 6 NICUs in Brazil, Couto and colleagues[57] demonstrated that 186 (64.1%) of 290 isolates of *K pneumoniae* were resistant to third-generation cephalosporins. Furthermore, it is estimated that 70% of *Klebsiella* spp blood stream infections in NICUs in developing countries are resistant to gentamicin.[58]

The impact of infection caused by antibiotic-resistant GNB has varied. Khassawneh and colleagues[59] reported a 30% crude mortality rate caused by highly resistant GNB; 48% of deaths occurred within the first 3 days of infection. However, Kristof and colleagues[60] found no statistically significant difference in mortality between infections caused by ESBL-producing and non–ESBL-producing *Klebsiella* spp (1 in 8 vs 1 in 37, respectively). Of note, Abdel-Hady and colleagues[61] found that infection with ESBL-producing *K pneumoniae* was associated with a 3-fold higher crude mortality. Costs attributable to AROs can be remarkable. An outbreak of ESBL-producing *K pneumoniae* consisting of 8 infected and 14 colonized infants cost nearly $350,000, mainly attributable to increased health care worker time and closed hospital beds.[62]

Invasive *Candida* spp infections are associated with an attributable mortality rate of 13% and are the third most frequent cause of late-onset sepsis in VLBW preterm neonates.[3,63] The burden of resistance is largely determined by the prevalent *Candida* spp; *Candida albicans* and *Candida parapsilosis* species are usually susceptible to fluconazole, whereas *Candida krusei* is intrinsically resistant to fluconazole. Of note, *Candida lusitaniae*, a relatively rare cause of candidemia, is intrinsically resistant to amphotericin. Although candidemia in adult and pediatric ICUs are increasingly caused by nonalbicans species,[64–66] this trend has not been noted in NICUs. From 1995 to 2004, there was no increase in the number of infections caused by *Candida glabrata* or *C krusei* in 128 American NICUs.[63] Although there are no data supporting the increased virulence of different *Candida* spp in NICU populations, speciation is critical to detect possible intrinsic resistance and susceptibility testing should be performed before treatment with fluconazole.

PREVENTION
Judicious Use of Antibiotics

Infants hospitalized in the NICU have high rates of antibiotic use. In a national point-prevalence study of 29 NICUs in the United States, 43% of patients in the NICU were receiving antimicrobials on the survey date.[67] Exposure to antibiotics is a risk factor for AROs; use of penicillin class agents have been associated with the emergence of MRSA,[68] and in the NICU, use of third-generation cephalosporin agents have been associated with the emergence of ESBL GNB as well as invasive candidiasis.[69,70]

Antimicrobial stewardship is increasingly being promoted as a means to limit AMR and improve quality of care. The Infectious Disease Society of America reviewed potential strategies to improve antimicrobial use and developed evidence-based recommendations for antimicrobial stewardship programs.[71] One of the hallmarks of successful antimicrobial stewardship programs has been the use of an interdisciplinary team. Such programs report the collaborative efforts of intensivists, infectious diseases physicians, nurses, pharmacists, hospital epidemiologists, and bioinformatics specialists. However, antimicrobial stewardship programs are not commonly used in pediatric settings.[72]

The Centers for Disease Control and Prevention has initiated a new program to combat the threat of antibiotic resistance in acute care settings. (Arjun Srinivasan, MD, Atlanta, GA, personal communication, March 2010). The program is called the

"Get Smart in Healthcare Settings: Know When Antibiotics Work" campaign and consists of 4 major concepts: timely antibiotic management; appropriate selection, administration, and de-escalation of antibiotics; access to infectious disease expertise; and improved data monitoring and transparency.

Although none of the evidence-based national antibiotic stewardship initiatives have been specifically developed for hospitalized infants, the general principles intended to improve antibiotic use are still applicable to the NICU population as shown in **Table 3**. Studies of biomarkers have shown that these principles are relevant; interleukin-8 and C-reactive protein have been successfully used to guide initiation of antibiotic therapy,[73,74] and procalcitonin has been used to guide duration of therapy.[75] Appropriate management of suspected infections can be improved by educational interventions stressing adequate blood culture volumes.[76] In the NICU, education about the antibiotic spectra of activity may improve antibiotic use because failure to de-escalate antibiotic coverage is often responsible for excessive antibiotic use.[77]

Interventions to improve antibiotic stewardship that use antibiotic restriction have been evaluated in neonatal populations. Restricting the use of cephalosporin agents

Table 3
Centers for Disease Control and Prevention principles for judicious antibiotic use: relevant NICU examples

"Get Smart" Principles	Examples for the NICU

Timely antibiotic management
  Accurately identify patients who need
    antibiotic therapy
  Obtain appropriate cultures before start of
    antibiotics
  Administer antibiotics promptly
	Use biomarkers such as CRP to guide
	  initiation of therapy
	Obtain simultaneous CVC and peripheral
	  blood cultures when possible
	Obtain sufficient blood culture volumes,
	  ie, >0.5 mL

Appropriate selection, administration, and
  de-escalation of therapy
  Make empiric choices based on local
    antibiograms
  Do not give therapy with overlapping
    activity
  Give the right dose and at right interval
  Stop therapy promptly if indicated by
    culture results
  Review and adjust antibiotics at all
    transitions of care
  Monitor for toxicity and adjust therapy
    accordingly
	Change vancomycin to oxacillin once
	  infection with MSSA is determined
	Aim for higher vancomycin troughs
	  (15–20 µg/mL) for suspected meningitis
	Discontinue postoperative prophylaxis after
	  48 h
	Avoid redundant anaerobic spectrum
	  coverage (eg, metronidazole and
	  piperacillin/tazobactam)

Access to expertise at point of care
  Develop and make available expertise in
    antibiotic use
  Ensure that expertise is available to all
    physicians at the point of care
	Develop an antimicrobial stewardship team
	  incorporating neonatology, clinical
	  pharmacy, hospital epidemiology
	  infectious diseases, and nursing services
	Obtain infectious diseases consultations

Improved data monitoring and transparency
  Monitor and feedback data regarding
    antibiotic use and adverse events
  Make data visible to interdisciplinary care
    team
	Provide NICU-specific antibiograms for
	  common pathogens
	Measure and feedback data on antibiotic
	  prescribing to neonatologists

Abbreviations: CRP, C-reactive protein; CVC, central venous catheter.

was associated with a reduction in colonization with multidrug-resistant GNB.[78] Decreasing vancomycin use was considered an important factor in controlling an outbreak of VRE.[49] In contrast, Toltzis and colleagues[79] compared monthly rotations of gentamicin, piperacillin-tazobactam, and ceftazidime with unrestricted physician choice for treatment of suspected neonatal sepsis and found no reduction in AMR, hospital-acquired infections, or mortality, although there was notable contamination between the groups.

Another strategy with the potential to increase AROs is the prophylactic use of antimicrobial agents. As mentioned, the prophylactic use of fluconazole has not been associated, thus far, with the emergence of resistance.[17] In a meta-analysis of systemic prophylactic vancomycin therapy (either as continuous low-dose infusion or intermittent therapy), the investigators concluded that there were insufficient data to ascertain the risks of developing AROs.[80] In a later study, prophylactic vancomycin-heparin lock reduced the incidence of central line–associated blood stream infections in high-risk neonates with long-term use of central catheters and was not associated with increased vancomycin resistance.[81] Although the risk of developing vancomycin resistance may be lower with locks, because of low serum concentrations, larger multicenter studies are needed to ascertain the long-term risks of this strategy.

Infection Control Strategies

As described earlier, acquisition of AROs can occur via selective pressure from antibiotics or from a reservoir harboring resistant pathogens. Potential reservoirs have been described for gram-negative pathogens as well as MRSA, which include infected or colonized infants in the NICU whose pathogens are transmitted via the hands of health care workers, colonized health care workers, vertical transmission or postnatal transmission from mothers, postnatal transmission from other family members, the contaminated health care environment, intrinsically (contaminated during manufacture) or extrinsically contaminated (contaminated during preparation) infusates, or parenteral nutrition.[82]

Numerous studies have addressed risk factors, some of which are modifiable, for infections caused by AROs. Risk factors for infections caused by MRSA have included low birth weight, kangaroo care, eye discharge, and MRSA colonization in an individual infant as well as overall MRSA colonization rate in the NICU.[83,84] Risk factors for ESBL-producing K pneumoniae infection have included mechanical ventilation, VLBW less than 1500 g, parenteral nutrition, and previous treatment with third-generation cephalosporins.[61,85]

Infection control strategies aimed at preventing acquisition and transmission are outlined in **Table 4**. In addition to education, accurate identification and surveillance for AROs are crucial. Clinical microbiology laboratories must have adequate resources for appropriate susceptibility testing and rapid notification of results. The Department of Infection Prevention and Control must have a surveillance plan in place, which includes strategies for outbreak investigations. Surveillance cultures for AROs should be implemented when epidemiologically indicated or if mandated by public health authorities. There are several strategies for targeted surveillance cultures as described in **Table 4**. Rigorous efforts to contain antibiotic-resistant pathogens must be implemented. Hand hygiene is obviously the cornerstone of such efforts, and use of personal protective equipment is also an evidence-based strategy aimed at preventing transmission.[82] The use of eradication strategies is only applicable for MRSA, and these strategies may need to involve multiple body sites to prevent recolonization.[27] Eradication of MRSA colonization should be considered for individual infants because

Table 4
Infection control strategies aimed at reducing acquisition and transmission of AMR pathogens

Major Infection Control Components	Specific Strategies for Controlling AMR Organisms	Implementation of Specific Strategies
Education	Ongoing education of interdisciplinary stake holders	Education of front-line staff, including new hires
Identification of antibiotic-resistant pathogens	Accurate microbiology laboratory strategies	Appropriate clinical cultures (when indicated) and access to molecular typing
	Rapid notification	Consider screening cultures for high-risk infants, eg, those transferred from other NICUs or hospitalized in close proximity to another infant infected or colonized with an ARO
	Judicious use of screening cultures and surveillance cultures for infants or NICU staff	Consider surveillance cultures for staff if outbreak not halted by conventional measures
	Monitoring ill staff and visitors	Written policies for staff and visitors (including mothers) who are suspected or documented with AROs
Surveillance for AMR pathogens	Daily monitoring for epidemiologically significant AROs, eg, MRSA and GNB resistant to third-generation cephalosporins	Develop electronic surveillance for microbiology laboratory data
		NICU-specific antibiogram
		Track and trend resistance patterns
Containment of antibiotic-resistant pathogens	Hand hygiene by staff and families	Readily available hand-hygiene products
		Observations of hand hygiene, including missed opportunities and staff feedback
		Adequate supplies of gowns and gloves
	Prompt initiation of contact precautions, ie, staff don gown and gloves	Observations of transmission precautions, including missed opportunities and staff feedback
	Environmental cleaning	Written policies for environmental cleaning, equipment cleaning (eg, isolettes and radiant warmers)
Eradication of potential reservoirs of AMR pathogens	Consider eradication of MRSA colonization via topical antibiotics (eg, mupirocin), topical disinfectants (eg, chlorhexidine bathing)	Targeted eradication strategies may be indicated for endemic or epidemic colonization.
		Monitor for mupirocin resistance
Prevention of progression from colonization to infection	Reducing risk of infections via central line bundles	Implementation of evidence-based practices for insertion and maintenance of central lines, including peripherally inserted central catheters
		Daily assessment for need for catheter and prompt removal of catheter when no longer required

the rate of progression to active disease can range from 18% to 80%.[86] If staff is linked to an outbreak and ongoing transmission of MRSA is demonstrated despite implementation of other infection control strategies, eradication of staff colonization may be indicated.[27] Finally, minimizing exposure to potentially modifiable risk factors such as central venous catheters should be implemented as described in **Table 4**.

REFERENCES

1. Institute of Medicine. 100 initial priority topics for comparative effectiveness research. Available at: http://www.iom.edu/~/media/Files/Report%20Files/2009/ComparativeEffectivenessResearchPriorities/Stand%20Alone%20List%20of%2020100%20CER%20Priorities%20-%20for%20web.ashx. Accessed May 13, 2010.
2. Benjamin DK Jr, Stoll BJ. Infection in late preterm infants [abstract x]. Clin Perinatol 2006;33(4):871–82.
3. Stoll BJ, Hansen N, Fanaroff AA, et al. Late-onset sepsis in very low birth weight neonates: the experience of the NICHD Neonatal Research Network. Pediatrics 2002;110(2 Pt 1):285–91.
4. Maragakis LL, Winkler A, Tucker MG, et al. Outbreak of multidrug-resistant *Serratia marcescens* infection in a neonatal intensive care unit. Infect Control Hosp Epidemiol 2008;29(5):418–23.
5. Anderson B, Nicholas S, Sprague B, et al. Molecular and descriptive epidemiology of multidrug-resistant Enterobacteriaceae in hospitalized infants. Infect Control Hosp Epidemiol 2008;29(3):250–5.
6. Carey AJ, Della-Latta P, Huard R, et al. Changes in the molecular epidemiological characteristics of methicillin-resistant *Staphylococcus aureus* in a neonatal intensive care unit. Infect Control Hosp Epidemiol 2010;31(6):613–9.
7. Mammina C, Di Carlo P, Cipolla D, et al. Surveillance of multidrug-resistant gram-negative bacilli in a neonatal intensive care unit: prominent role of cross transmission. Am J Infect Control 2007;35(4):222–30.
8. Milisavljevic V, Wu F, Cimmotti J, et al. Genetic relatedness of *Staphylococcus epidermidis* from infected infants and staff in the neonatal intensive care unit. Am J Infect Control 2005;33(6):341–7.
9. Cimiotti JP, Haas JP, Della-Latta P, et al. Prevalence and clinical relevance of *Staphylococcus warneri* in the neonatal intensive care unit. Infect Control Hosp Epidemiol 2007;28(3):326–30.
10. Chen KT, Huard RC, Della-Latta P, et al. Prevalence of methicillin-sensitive and methicillin-resistant *Staphylococcus aureus* in pregnant women. Obstet Gynecol 2006;108(3 Pt 1):482–7.
11. Singh N, Leger MM, Campbell J, et al. Control of vancomycin-resistant enterococci in the neonatal intensive care unit. Infect Control Hosp Epidemiol 2005; 26(7):646–9.
12. Smith A, Saiman L, Zhou J, et al. Concordance of gastrointestinal tract colonization and subsequent bloodstream infections with gram-negative bacilli in very low birth-weight infants in the neonatal intensive care unit. Pediatr Infect Dis J 2010. [Epub ahead of print].
13. Toltzis P, Dul MJ, Hoyen C, et al. Molecular epidemiology of antibiotic-resistant gram-negative bacilli in a neonatal intensive care unit during a nonoutbreak period. Pediatrics 2001;108(5):1143–8.
14. Gupta A, Della-Latta P, Todd B, et al. Outbreak of extended-spectrum beta-lactamase-producing *Klebsiella pneumoniae* in a neonatal intensive care unit linked to artificial nails. Infect Control Hosp Epidemiol 2004;25(3):210–5.

15. Pitout JD, Laupland KB. Extended-spectrum beta-lactamase-producing Entero-bacteriaceae: an emerging public-health concern. Lancet Infect Dis 2008;8(3): 159–66.
16. Hawkey PM, Jones AM. The changing epidemiology of resistance. J Antimicrob Chemother 2009;64(Suppl 1):i3–10.
17. Manzoni P, Stolfi I, Pugni L, et al. A multicenter, randomized trial of prophylactic fluconazole in preterm neonates. N Engl J Med 2007;356(24):2483–95.
18. Kaufman D, Boyle R, Hazen KC, et al. Fluconazole prophylaxis against fungal colonization and infection in preterm infants. N Engl J Med 2001;345(23):1660–6.
19. Long SS, Stevenson DK. Reducing Candida infections during neonatal intensive care: management choices, infection control, and fluconazole prophylaxis. J Pediatr 2005;147(2):135–41.
20. Odds FC, Brown AJ, Gow NA. Antifungal agents: mechanisms of action. Trends Microbiol 2003;11(6):272–9.
21. Livermore DM, Hope R, Mushtaq S, et al. Orthodox and unorthodox clavulanate combinations against extended-spectrum beta-lactamase producers. Clin Micro-biol Infect 2008;14(Suppl 1):189–93.
22. Carey AJ, Saiman L, Polin RA. Hospital-acquired infections in the NICU: epidemi-ology for the new millennium. Clin Perinatol 2008;35(1):223–49, x.
23. Howden BP, Davies JK, Johnson PD, et al. Reduced vancomycin susceptibility in *Staphylococcus aureus*, including vancomycin-intermediate and heterogeneous vancomycin-intermediate strains: resistance mechanisms, laboratory detection, and clinical implications. Clin Microbiol Rev 23(1):99–139.
24. Rice LB. Antimicrobial resistance in gram-positive bacteria. Am J Med 2006; 119(6 Suppl 1):S11–9 [discussion: S62–70].
25. Regev-Yochay G, Rubinstein E, Barzilai A, et al. Methicillin-resistant *Staphylo-coccus aureus* in neonatal intensive care unit. Emerg Infect Dis 2005;11(3):453–6.
26. Haddad Q, Sobayo EI, Basit OB, et al. Outbreak of methicillin-resistant *Staphylo-coccus aureus* in a neonatal intensive care unit. J Hosp Infect 1993;23(3):211–22.
27. Carey AJ, Duchon J, Della-Latta P, et al. The epidemiology of methicillin-susceptible and methicillin-resistant *Staphylococcus aureus* in a neonatal inten-sive care unit, 2000–2007. J Perinatol 2010;30(2):135–9.
28. Bertin ML, Vinski J, Schmitt S, et al. Outbreak of methicillin-resistant *Staphylo-coccus aureus* colonization and infection in a neonatal intensive care unit epide-miologically linked to a healthcare worker with chronic otitis. Infect Control Hosp Epidemiol 2006;27(6):581–5.
29. Gerber SI, Jones RC, Scott MV, et al. Management of outbreaks of methicillin-resistant *Staphylococcus aureus* infection in the neonatal intensive care unit: a consensus statement. Infect Control Hosp Epidemiol 2006;27(2):139–45.
30. Cohen-Wolkowiez M, Benjamin DK Jr, Fowler VG Jr, et al. Mortality and neurode-velopmental outcome after *Staphylococcus aureus* bacteremia in infants. Pediatr Infect Dis J 2007;26(12):1159–61.
31. de Hoog M, Mouton JW, van den Anker JN. Vancomycin: pharmacokinetics and administration regimens in neonates. Clin Pharmacokinet 2004;43(7):417–40.
32. Centers for Disease Control and Prevention (CDC). Community-associated methicillin-resistant *Staphylococcus aureus* infection among healthy newborns–Chicago and Los Angeles County, 2004. MMWR Morb Mortal Wkly Rep 2006; 55(12):329–32.
33. McAdams RM, Ellis MW, Trevino S, et al. Spread of methicillin-resistant *Staphylo-coccus aureus* USA300 in a neonatal intensive care unit. Pediatr Int 2008;50(6): 810–5.

34. Healy CM, Hulten KG, Palazzi DL, et al. Emergence of new strains of methicillin-resistant *Staphylococcus aureus* in a neonatal intensive care unit. Clin Infect Dis 2004;39(10):1460–6.
35. Kuint J, Barzilai A, Regev-Yochay G, et al. Comparison of community-acquired methicillin-resistant *Staphylococcus aureus* bacteremia to other staphylococcal species in a neonatal intensive care unit. Eur J Pediatr 2007;166(4):319–25.
36. Fortunov RM, Hulten KG, Hammerman WA, et al. Community-acquired *Staphylococcus aureus* infections in term and near-term previously healthy neonates. Pediatrics 2006;118(3):874–81.
37. Krediet TG, Jones ME, Janssen K, et al. Prevalence of molecular types and mecA gene carriage of coagulase-negative Staphylococci in a neonatal intensive care unit: relation to nosocomial septicemia. J Clin Microbiol 2001;39(9):3376–8.
38. Krediet TG, Mascini EM, van Rooij E, et al. Molecular epidemiology of coagulase-negative staphylococci causing sepsis in a neonatal intensive care unit over an 11-year period. J Clin Microbiol 2004;42(3):992–5.
39. Klingenberg C, Ronnestad A, Anderson AS, et al. Persistent strains of coagulase-negative staphylococci in a neonatal intensive care unit: virulence factors and invasiveness. Clin Microbiol Infect 2007;13(11):1100–11.
40. Center KJ, Reboli AC, Hubler R, et al. Decreased vancomycin susceptibility of coagulase-negative staphylococci in a neonatal intensive care unit: evidence of spread of *Staphylococcus warneri*. J Clin Microbiol 2003;41(10):4660–5.
41. Van Der Zwet WC, Debets-Ossenkopp YJ, Reinders E, et al. Nosocomial spread of a *Staphylococcus capitis* strain with heteroresistance to vancomycin in a neonatal intensive care unit. J Clin Microbiol 2002;40(7):2520–5.
42. Villari P, Sarnataro C, Iacuzio L. Molecular epidemiology of *Staphylococcus epidermidis* in a neonatal intensive care unit over a three-year period. J Clin Microbiol 2000;38(5):1740–6.
43. Graham PL, Ampofo K, Saiman L. Linezolid treatment of vancomycin-resistant *Enterococcus faecium* ventriculitis. Pediatr Infect Dis J 2002;21(8):798–800.
44. Ang JY, Lua JL, Turner DR, et al. Vancomycin-resistant *Enterococcus faecium* endocarditis in a premature infant successfully treated with linezolid. Pediatr Infect Dis J 2003;22(12):1101–3.
45. Borgmann S, Niklas DM, Klare I, et al. Two episodes of vancomycin-resistant *Enterococcus faecium* outbreaks caused by two genetically different clones in a newborn intensive care unit. Int J Hyg Environ Health 2004;207(4):386–9.
46. Kumar S, Kohlhoff S, Valencia G, et al. Treatment of vancomycin-resistant *Enterococcus faecium* ventriculitis in a neonate. Int J Antimicrob Agents 2007;29(6):740–1.
47. Lee HK, Lee WG, Cho SR. Clinical and molecular biological analysis of a nosocomial outbreak of vancomycin-resistant enterococci in a neonatal intensive care unit. Acta Paediatr 1999;88(6):651–4.
48. McNeeley DF, Saint-Louis F, Noel GJ. Neonatal enterococcal bacteremia: an increasingly frequent event with potentially untreatable pathogens. Pediatr Infect Dis J 1996;15(9):800–5.
49. Rupp ME, Marion N, Fey PD, et al. Outbreak of vancomycin-resistant *Enterococcus faecium* in a neonatal intensive care unit. Infect Control Hosp Epidemiol 2001;22(5):301–3.
50. Duchon J, Graham Iii P, Della-Latta P, et al. Epidemiology of enterococci in a neonatal intensive care unit. Infect Control Hosp Epidemiol 2008;29(4):374–6.

51. Stoll BJ, Hansen NI, Higgins RD, et al. Very low birth weight preterm infants with early onset neonatal sepsis: the predominance of gram-negative infections continues in the National Institute of Child Health and Human Development Neonatal Research Network, 2002–2003. Pediatr Infect Dis J 2005; 24(7):635–9.
52. Nambiar S, Singh N. Change in epidemiology of health care-associated infections in a neonatal intensive care unit. Pediatr Infect Dis J 2002;21(9): 839–42.
53. Townsend SM, Hurrell E, Caubilla-Barron J, et al. Characterization of an extended-spectrum beta-lactamase *Enterobacter hormaechei* nosocomial outbreak, and other *Enterobacter hormaechei* misidentified as *Cronobacter* (*Enterobacter*) *sakazakii*. Microbiology 2008;154(Pt 12):3659–67.
54. Sehgal R, Gaind R, Chellani H, et al. Extended-spectrum beta lactamase-producing gram-negative bacteria: clinical profile and outcome in a neonatal intensive care unit. Ann Trop Paediatr 2007;27(1):45–54.
55. Jeena P, Thompson E, Nchabeleng M, et al. Emergence of multi-drug-resistant *Acinetobacter anitratus* species in neonatal and paediatric intensive care units in a developing country: concern about antimicrobial policies. Ann Trop Paediatr 2001;21(3):245–51.
56. Singh N, Patel KM, Leger MM, et al. Risk of resistant infections with Enterobacteriaceae in hospitalized neonates. Pediatr Infect Dis J 2002;21(11):1029–33.
57. Couto RC, Carvalho EA, Pedrosa TM, et al. A 10-year prospective surveillance of nosocomial infections in neonatal intensive care units. Am J Infect Control 2007; 35(3):183–9.
58. Zaidi AK, Huskins WC, Thaver D, et al. Hospital-acquired neonatal infections in developing countries. Lancet 2005;365(9465):1175–88.
59. Khassawneh M, Khader Y, Abuqtaish N. Clinical features of neonatal sepsis caused by resistant Gram-negative bacteria. Pediatr Int 2009;51(3):332–6.
60. Kristof K, Szabo D, Marsh JW, et al. Extended-spectrum beta-lactamase-producing Klebsiella spp. in a neonatal intensive care unit: risk factors for the infection and the dynamics of the molecular epidemiology. Eur J Clin Microbiol Infect Dis 2007;26(8):563–70.
61. Abdel-Hady H, Hawas S, El-Daker M, et al. Extended-spectrum beta-lactamase producing *Klebsiella pneumoniae* in neonatal intensive care unit. J Perinatol 2008;28(10):685–90.
62. Stone PW, Gupta A, Loughrey M, et al. Attributable costs and length of stay of an extended-spectrum beta-lactamase-producing *Klebsiella pneumoniae* outbreak in a neonatal intensive care unit. Infect Control Hosp Epidemiol 2003;24(8):601–6.
63. Fridkin SK, Kaufman D, Edwards JR, et al. Changing incidence of Candida bloodstream infections among NICU patients in the United States: 1995–2004. Pediatrics 2006;117(5):1680–7.
64. Wisplinghoff H, Bischoff T, Tallent SM, et al. Nosocomial bloodstream infections in US hospitals: analysis of 24,179 cases from a prospective nationwide surveillance study. Clin Infect Dis 2004;39(3):309–17.
65. Pappas PG, Rex JH, Lee J, et al. A prospective observational study of candidemia: epidemiology, therapy, and influences on mortality in hospitalized adult and pediatric patients. Clin Infect Dis 2003;37(5):634–43.
66. Neu N, Malik M, Lunding A, et al. Epidemiology of candidemia at a children's hospital, 2002 to 2006. Pediatr Infect Dis J 2009;28(9):806–9.

67. Grohskopf LA, Huskins WC, Sinkowitz-Cochran RL, et al. Use of antimicrobial agents in United States neonatal and pediatric intensive care patients. Pediatr Infect Dis J 2005;24(9):766–73.
68. Muller A, Mauny F, Talon D, et al. Effect of individual- and group-level antibiotic exposure on MRSA isolation: a multilevel analysis. J Antimicrob Chemother 2006;58(4):878–81.
69. Zaoutis TE, Goyal M, Chu JH, et al. Risk factors for and outcomes of bloodstream infection caused by extended-spectrum beta-lactamase-producing *Escherichia coli* and Klebsiella species in children. Pediatrics 2005;115(4):942–9.
70. Cotten CM, McDonald S, Stoll B, et al. The association of third-generation cephalosporin use and invasive candidiasis in extremely low birth-weight infants. Pediatrics 2006;118(2):717–22.
71. Dellit TH, Owens RC, McGowan JE Jr, et al. Infectious Diseases Society of America and the Society for Healthcare Epidemiology of America guidelines for developing an institutional program to enhance antimicrobial stewardship. Clin Infect Dis 2007;44(2):159–77.
72. Hersh AL, Beekmann SE, Polgreen PM, et al. Antimicrobial stewardship programs in pediatrics. Infect Control Hosp Epidemiol 2009;30(12):1211–7.
73. Franz AR, Bauer K, Schalk A, et al. Measurement of interleukin 8 in combination with C-reactive protein reduced unnecessary antibiotic therapy in newborn infants: a multicenter, randomized, controlled trial. Pediatrics 2004;114(1):1–8.
74. Ehl S, Gering B, Bartmann P, et al. C-reactive protein is a useful marker for guiding duration of antibiotic therapy in suspected neonatal bacterial infection. Pediatrics 1997;99(2):216–21.
75. Stocker M, Fontana M, El Helou S, et al. Use of procalcitonin-guided decision-making to shorten antibiotic therapy in suspected neonatal early-onset sepsis: prospective randomized intervention trial. Neonatology. 97(2):165–174.
76. Connell TG, Rele M, Cowley D, et al. How reliable is a negative blood culture result? Volume of blood submitted for culture in routine practice in a children's hospital. Pediatrics 2007;119(5):891–6.
77. Patel SJ, Oshodi A, Prasad P, et al. Antibiotic use in neonatal intensive care units and adherence with Centers for Disease Control and Prevention 12 Step Campaign to Prevent Antimicrobial Resistance. Pediatr Infect Dis J 2009; 28(12):1047–51.
78. Calil R, Marba ST, von Nowakonski A, et al. Reduction in colonization and nosocomial infection by multiresistant bacteria in a neonatal unit after institution of educational measures and restriction in the use of cephalosporins. Am J Infect Control 2001;29(3):133–8.
79. Toltzis P, Dul MJ, Hoyen C, et al. The effect of antibiotic rotation on colonization with antibiotic-resistant bacilli in a neonatal intensive care unit. Pediatrics 2002; 110(4):707–11.
80. Craft AP, Finer NN, Barrington KJ. Vancomycin for prophylaxis against sepsis in preterm neonates. Cochrane Database Syst Rev 2000;2:CD001971.
81. Garland JS, Alex CP, Henrickson KJ, et al. A vancomycin-heparin lock solution for prevention of nosocomial bloodstream infection in critically ill neonates with peripherally inserted central venous catheters: a prospective, randomized trial. Pediatrics 2005;116(2):e198–205.
82. Siegel JD, Rhinehart E, Jackson M, et al. 2007 guideline for isolation precautions: preventing transmission of infectious agents in health care settings. Am J Infect Control 2007;35(10 Suppl 2):S65–164.

83. Sakaki H, Nishioka M, Kanda K, et al. An investigation of the risk factors for infection with methicillin-resistant *Staphylococcus aureus* among patients in a neonatal intensive care unit. Am J Infect Control 2009;37(7):580–6.
84. Huang YC, Chou YH, Su LH, et al. Methicillin-resistant *Staphylococcus aureus* colonization and its association with infection among infants hospitalized in neonatal intensive care units. Pediatrics 2006;118(2):469–74.
85. Huang Y, Zhuang S, Du M. Risk factors of nosocomial infection with extended-spectrum beta-lactamase-producing bacteria in a neonatal intensive care unit in China. Infection 2007;35(5):339–45.
86. Bizzarro MJ, Gallagher PG. Antibiotic-resistant organisms in the neonatal intensive care unit. Semin Perinatol 2007;31(1):26–32.

New Concepts of Microbial Translocation in the Neonatal Intestine: Mechanisms and Prevention

Michael P. Sherman, MD

KEYWORDS

• Intestinal microbiota
• Enterocytes, goblet cells, and Paneth cells
• Lactoferrin, probiotics, and prebiotics

In very low-birth-weight (VLBW) (<1500 g) infants, late-onset neonatal sepsis and necrotizing enterocolitis (NEC) prolong the hospital stay, increase the cost of care, and place infants at greater risk for morbidity and mortality.[1] Long-term follow-up studies have demonstrated that these infections significantly increase the risk of neurologic disabilities.[2] With incidences of approximately 20% and 5% to 10%, respectively, late-onset sepsis (LOS) and NEC in VLBW infants need new preventive approaches. A long-held belief is that LOS and NEC result from bacterial translocation (BT). Bacterial translocation is defined as invasion of indigenous intestinal bacteria through the mucosa into normally sterile tissue.[3] This definition has been extended to include bacterial toxins or antigens, which damage intestinal epithelia and enter the circulation, resulting in a systemic inflammatory response.[4] Local BT through the intestinal mucosa or toxin-related injury of intestinal epithelia is associated with NEC,[5] whereas BT beyond the intestine causes sepsis and multiorgan failure.[6,7] This article describes (1) development of the intestinal microbiota, (2) how immaturity of the nascent epithelial lining of the gastrointestinal (GI) tract and its submucosal tissues mediate BT, (3) strategies to accelerate barrier functions in the immature GI tract, and (4) the effects of nutrition and colonization by commensal bacteria on the susceptibility of the immature intestine to BT.

This research was supported by NIH grant R44 HD057744 and a Gerber Foundation grant.
University of Missouri, Department of Child Health, Children's Hospital, 404 Keene Street, Neonatology Suite 206, Columbia, MO 65201, USA
E-mail address: ShermanMP@health.missouri.edu

Clin Perinatol 37 (2010) 565–579
doi:10.1016/j.clp.2010.05.006
0095-5108/10/$ – see front matter © 2010 Elsevier Inc. All rights reserved.

EMERGENCE OF INTESTINAL MICROBIOTA AFTER BIRTH
General Principles

Healthy term infants stay with their mothers, breastfeed, and acquire intestinal micro-flora from the mother that is genetically compatible. This theory, espoused by Hooper and colleagues,[8] holds that proper postnatal acquisition of genetically compatible gut microbiota improves nutrition and fortifies the gut's epithelial barrier. In contrast, VLBW infants are almost always separated from their mothers and are cared for in a neonatal ICU containing resistant and invasive pathogens. Although early and full human milk feedings reduce LOS,[9] this goal is difficult to achieve.

Dysbiosis of the intestine, or abnormal gut flora, increases the risk of LOS and NEC in VLBW infants. Reasons for dysbiosis include birth by cesarean section, hygiene practices, prolonged antibiotic administration, reduced bowel motility, immature epithelial host defenses, type or mode of nutrition, and parenteral nutrition.[10–12] Strategies that alter these variables reduce the risk of LOS and NEC.[12]

Defining an Intestinal Microflora in Neonates that Causes Bacterial Translocation

Standard bacteriologic culture techniques have traditionally been used to define the acquisition and succession of bacteria in the immature intestine. *Escherichia coli*, staphylococci, and enterococci are present in neonatal stools within days of birth, whereas the genera *Bifidobacterium*, *Clostridium*, and *Bacteroides* can be detected within a week or two.[10,13] This is also the time period when NEC becomes prevalent. In 1974, Hill and colleagues[14] showed that BT was associated with an epidemic of sepsis, meningitis, and NEC due to *Klebsiella*. *Klebsiella*, and the hydrogen sulfide gas this microbe produces during fermentation, were found during micropuncture of the cysts in infants who had pneumatosis intestinalis. Other studies have shown that δ-toxin produced by staphylococci can disrupt gut epithelia and initiate bacter-emia and NEC.[15,16] Many studies identifying multiple microorganisms in infants with NEC and LOS highlight the difficulty in defining a disease-specific bacterial pathogen.

Non–culture-based microbial analyses of feces are currently being used to under-stand the bacterial pathogenesis of NEC.[17–19] de la Cochetière and colleagues[20] iso-lated DNA from stool, amplified microbial 16S ribosomal DNA, and then used temporal temperature gradient gel electrophoresis of the polymerase chain reaction (PCR) amplicons for identification. In three infants who developed NEC (but in none of the control infants), *Clostridium perfringens* was identified. Causation could not be linked, however, to the presence of *Clostridium*. Wang and colleagues[21] studied 10 preterm infants with NEC (and 10 matched controls) using DNA isolated from feces that was amplified using PCR and subjected to terminal-restriction fragment length polymor-phism analysis. A sequence library of 16S rRNA for enteric bacteria was used for iden-tification. Patients with NEC had less bacterial diversity and an increased abundance of γ-proteobacteria (eg, *E coli*) in the stools. In contrast, a recent study by Mshvildadze and colleagues[22] using pyrosequencing technology demonstrated that the overall microbial profiles in patients with NEC were not different from those of control infants. Thus, to date, molecular methods have not clarified the bacterial pathogenesis in NEC. It is possible that NEC may be similar to Crohn disease wherein the enteric bacterial community host genetics, and defects in immunity, in combination, contribute to path-ogenesis.[23] Molecular techniques for microbe identification (metagenomics) will not delineate (1) high numbers of diverse, infectious bacteria attacking gut epithelia (microbial load), (2) multiple mechanisms used by pathogens to gain entry into or around intestinal epithelia (virulence), or (3) bacterial toxins that cause necrotic or apoptotic death of intestinal lining cells (lethality).[24] Combining molecular microbial identification in patients with NEC with knowledge from the human microbiome project,[25] however, may enable researchers and caregivers to better understand the connection between BT and NEC.

Microbe and Epithelial Cell Interactions that Mediate Bacterial Translocation

As shown in **Fig. 1**, bacteria reach the submucosa of the intestine via transcellular and paracellular pathways, whereas microbial toxins leave the intestinal lumen via the paracellular pathway after loss of tight junctions between enterocytes. Most neonatal studies of BT have been performed in vitro,[26] and in vivo information about BT in the immature intestine is limited.[27] Understanding of bacteria and enterocyte interactions that initiate BT is largely derived from studies of enteropathogenic, enteroinvasive, and enterohemorrhagic *E coli*, *Shigella* spp, *Salmonella* spp, *Listeria monocytogenes*, and *Yersinia* spp.[27–29]

Several mechanisms of BT have been identified. A zipper mechanism is used by *Listeria monocytogenes* and *Yersinia pseudotuberculosis* to enter enterocytes, whereas *Shigella* and *Salmonella* use a trigger mechanism for transcytosis.[29] The zipper mechanism exploits transmembrane cell-adhesion proteins as receptors for the bacteria. The trigger mechanism uses the bacterial type III secretory system, which involves a bacterial needle-like probe that injects dedicated bacterial effectors into epithelia and the injected molecules modify the cytoskeleton to facilitate bacterial entry. Other adhesive mechanisms allow invasive *E coli* to bind to epithelial surfaces and enter enterocytes while also initiating inflammation.[30–32] During inflammation, production of nitric oxide alters expression and localization of the tight junction zonulin proteins, ZO-1, ZO-2, ZO-3, and occludin.[33] Disruption of tight junctions that surround the upper part and lateral surfaces of enterocytes leads to intestinal hyperpermeability and

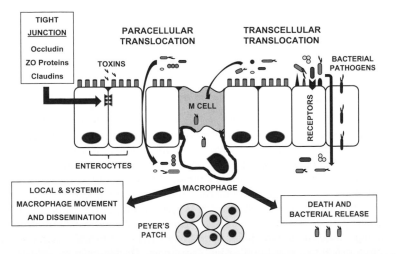

Fig. 1. Mechanisms of BT in the small intestine. Multiple pathways, receptors, and cells are involved in BT from the intestinal lumen. Toxins, such as flagellin, endotoxins, and exotoxins, and other bacterial products can disrupt tight junctions and facilitate paracellular translocation of bacteria between intestinal epithelial cells. Transcellular translocation of bacteria can occur via receptors, including intelectin (also LF receptor), type III secretory system, Toll-like receptors, LFA-1 (lectin) receptor, β1 integrin, and IgA, displayed on M cells. Bacterial uptake through these cells can result in systemic dissemination of the microbe.

predisposes to BT. *Cronobacter* spp (*Enterobacter sakazaki*) requires the host cell cytoskeleton for transcytosis, a process enhanced by disruption of tight junctions.[34,35] Toll-like receptors (TLRs) are present on the luminal surface of enterocytes to sense danger and activate host defenses, but TLRs can also be harmful by mediating phagocytosis and translocation of bacteria across the intestinal barrier.[36] Finally, the enteric bacterial community plays a role in BT as evidenced by a study showing *Campylobacter jejuni* assisting commensal bacteria to cross gut epithelia using lipid rafts.[37]

Once pathogens pass the mucus and epithelial barriers, submucosal macrophages ingest translocated bacteria. This process occurs without initiation of an inflammatory response.[38] The efferent vagus nerve enhances intestinal macrophage phagocytic activity by stimulating the α4-β2 nicotinic acetylcholine receptor.[39] The vagus nerve also dampens cytokine-driven inflammation via its actions on the α7 nicotinic acetylcholine receptor on intestinal macrophages in a process termed, *the cholinergic anti-inflammatory pathway*.[40–42] The physiology of intestinal macrophages and the efferent vagal regulatory system in the intestine of neonates has not been characterized. If intestinal macrophages are dysfunctional in VLBW infants, as they are in adults with Crohn disease,[43] this dysfunction may contribute to BT. Pathogenic bacteria can readily destroy submucosal macrophages, thereby enhancing BT.

A major task of submucosal macrophages is protection from BT that occurs via microfold epithelium over Peyer patches (called M cells).[44] M cells evaluate the intestinal lumen environment and transport bacteria through the epithelial barrier to submucosal macrophages and dendritic cells, which then act as antigen-presenting cells. M cells are portals for BT because they have no peptide antibiotic defense akin to enterocytes and they are not covered by a mucin layer. Dendritic cells use secretory IgA (sIgA) to take up bacteria from M cells.[45] Pathogen-specific sIgA secretion into the neonatal gut lumen occurs over time in relation to antigen exposure; thus, at birth, sIgA is not secreted into the bowel to protect against BT. Neonates can, however, passively acquire sIgA from maternal breast milk.

GUT EPITHELIA AND PROTECTION AGAINST BACTERIAL TRANSLOCATION

The mechanisms used by goblet cells, enterocytes, and Paneth cells to protect VLBW infants from BT are summarized in **Table 1**.[46–66]

The Nonepithelial Barrier

The first line of defense for preventing BT is the mucous coat overlying gut epithelia, produced by goblet cells. There are misconceptions about the mucus layer because histologic preparations have not delineated its true characteristics.[46] The mucus layer is now appreciated as a gel-like diphasic system that exists in a liquid phase near the lumen and a more solid phase near the epithelia. The outer or luminal mucus layer has degraded mucin, diluted antimicrobial peptides, and some bacteria. The epithelium-associated mucus layer is firmly bound, is rich in natural antibiotic peptides, and has a sterile microaerobic environment. In the crypts, antimicrobial peptide concentrations are high because of Paneth cell secretions. Paneth cells are in close proximity to and serve a protective role for intestinal stem cells. Goblet cells secrete MUC2 and trefoil factors to facilitate mucin polymerization. MUC2 is the structural component of the protective mucus layer, whereas trefoil factors serve important protective roles, such as prevention of enterocyte apoptosis and renewal of epithelial cells. MUC2 is synthesized rapidly in preterm infants based on threonine incorporation into its peptide backbone.[54] MUC2 mRNA appears at 12 weeks of human gestation in the jejunum, ileum, and colon.[55] In newborn animals, the mucus layer is said to be

Table 1
Functional characteristics of goblet cells, enterocytes, and Paneth cells

Immunologic Agent	Cell Type	Regulation	Function
Mucin (MUC2)	Goblet cells Paneth cells	Constitutive; stimulation via TLR ligands, cytokines, growth factors/hormones	Hydrophilic mucus, physical barrier, lubrication
Trefoil peptides	Goblet cells	Constitutive	Mucin polymerization, antiapoptotic, epithelial renewal
Antimicrobial peptides: α-defensins Secretory Phospholipase A_2 Lysozyme Angiogenin 4 Cathelicidins α-defensins	Paneth cells Paneth cells Paneth cells Paneth cells Enterocytes Enterocytes	Constitutive, stimulation via TLR or NOD ligands; cholinergic stimulation releases microbicides	Disrupt microbial walls, promote inflammation
Lectins RegIIIγ, collectins	Paneth cells and enterocytes	Constitutive, stimulation via TLR ligands	Antimicrobial activity
Protease inhibitors: Secretory leukocyte protease inhibitor Elafin	Paneth cells and enterocytes	Constitutive	Antimicrobial activity
Phospholipids	Enterocytes	Cortisone	Lubricant in mucus
Nucleotide-binding oligomerization domain	Enterocyte—NOD1 Paneth cell—NOD2	Constitutive	Microbial sensors, activate inflammation

discontinuous, which would promote BT; however, there is speculation that this finding could be an artifact. The quality and quantity of mucin in preterm infants are not well characterized.

The Epithelial Barrier

Gut epithelia are essential to host defense in the distal ileum and proximal colon, which are the primary areas of involvement in NEC.[56] **Fig. 2** illustrates how Paneth cells sense commensal microflora, leading to release of angiogenins that mediate development of the epithelia and villi.[57] Goblet cells secrete the mucus barrier, a primary defense against BT. Enterocytes also serve as multifunctional protectors of the gut barrier. Originating from stem cells at the base of the crypts, enterocytes migrate toward the villus tip.[47] Human enterocytes contain β-defensins that are secreted into the mucus layer and defend against bacterial transcytosis.[48] If enterocytes are invaded, these defensins are secreted and act as chemoattractants for dendritic cells and T cells. Cathelicidins, including LL-37/CAP18 and CRAMP, are a second class of antimicrobial peptides in enterocytes which are microbicidal for gram-positive and gram-negative bacteria.[49] LL-37 has chemotactic activity for monocytes, macrophages, and T cells and initiates Th1-related cytokine secretion by dendritic cells.

Paneth cells, epithelia localized to the crypts of Lieberkühn, contribute significantly to gut innate immunity. Mallow and colleagues[58] used in situ hybridization to localize

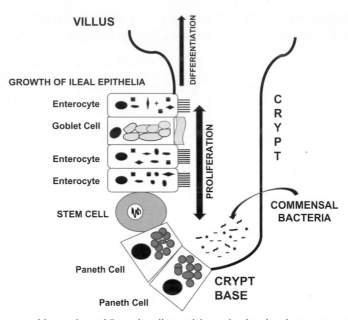

Fig. 2. Commensal bacteria and Paneth cells participate in the development, maintenance, and repair of an intestinal villus. Stem cells at the base of the crypts give rise to four cell lineages (enterocytes, goblet cells, Paneth cells, and intestinal neuroendocrine epithelia). These cells participate in host defense against bacterial translocation.[51,57] The role of neuroendocrine epithelia in host defense of the intestinal villus is undefined.

α-defensins to Paneth cells during human gestation. At 19 to 24 weeks of gestation, mRNA levels of α-defensins in the small intestine are 40- to 250- fold lower than that seen in adults. A reduced number of Paneth cells per crypt at 24 weeks of gestation, compared with that in adults, may partly explain the lower mRNA levels of α-defensins. In contrast, Paneth cells in intestinal segments obtained from infants with NEC exhibit increased mRNA transcripts for α-defensins.[59] This is a late finding, and it may simply imply that bacterial pathogens induce expression of α-defensins. Coutinho and colleagues[60] demonstrated a depletion of lysozyme in Paneth cells in infants with NEC. Further support for the importance of Paneth cells in neonatal host defense comes from studies using dithizone to selectively kill Paneth cells and reduce their antimicrobial granules.[61] When neonatal rats were given dithizone and then infected with enteroinvasive *E coli*, all pups developed bacteremia caused by *E coli* and some animals developed ileal necrosis akin to NEC.[61] Studies of neonatal mice with a genetic gain or loss of α-defensins (cryptdins) indicate that these Paneth cell–associated antimicrobial peptides play a role in the emergence of the intestinal microbiota after birth.[62] The pathogenesis of Crohn disease is also linked to a deficiency of α-defensins.[63] Finally, cortisone increases the number and complexity of Paneth cells in neonatal rats,[64] and antenatal steroids are linked to a reduction in NEC in preterm infants.[65] Taken together, these data support the important role of Paneth cells in modulating enteric bacteria and in serving as a major innate defense against BT, LOS, and NEC in preterm infants.[50]

Paneth cells have additional roles beyond prevention of BT,[51–53] such as sensing changes in the microflora of the mature gut and maintaining host-microbial homeostasis at the mucosal surface.[66] Paneth cells also stimulate blood vessel growth during development and after intestinal injury, via production of angiogenins.[57,66] Paneth cells produce and respond to inflammation-modulating cytokines. They have abundant mRNA transcripts for tumor necrosis factor α (TNF-α) and there is a marked increase in TNF-α mRNA in Paneth cells in infants with eosinophil- and macrophage-related infiltrates observed during NEC.[67] Although some evidence suggests that TNF-α from Paneth cells may be responsible for the massive necrosis seen during NEC, other researchers have observed that TNF-α is involved in villus repair after injury. Other cytokines have been reported to regulate Paneth cell number and function. For example, the combination of IL-9 and IL-13 was shown to mediate Paneth cell hyperplasia and up-regulate innate immunity at the gut's epithelial barrier.[68]

THE ROLE OF NUTRITION IN PREVENTING BACTERIAL TRANSLOCATION
General Principles

During the third trimester of pregnancy, the fetus swallows nutrient-, growth factor-, and antibiotic peptide–rich amniotic fluid.[69] Human milk is even more complex than amniotic fluid, and it continues to enhance intestinal development after birth.[70] In addition to its nutrient composition, human milk contains hormones, growth factors, cytokines, immunomodulators, natural peptide antibiotics, sIgA, and probiotic bacteria.[70–76] sIgA in milk is the end result of crosstalk between the mother and her environmental microbiota.[76] The continuum of drinking amniotic fluid and then human milk results in NEC being infrequent in breastfed infants born at term gestation. VLBW infants are born without proper maturation of the intestine or its innate antimicrobial defenses, and mother's milk is the fallback mechanism to prevent BT, LOS, or NEC. A recent report reaffirms that an exclusive human milk diet, rather than partial or full bovine milk-based nutrition, significantly reduces the incidence of NEC.[77] VLBW infants cannot consume enough breast milk early in life to achieve an adequate innate host defense in the immature intestine. To address the lack of mother's milk after birth, lactoferrin (LF), probiotics, and prebiotics are being fed to VLBW infants with the goal of boosting innate host defenses against BT, LOS, and NEC.

Lactoferrin for Prevention of Bacterial Translocation in Infants

LF is a member of the transferrin family and a multifunctional protein with high concentrations in colostrum and a stable content in mature milk. As summarized in **Table 2**, LF has antimicrobial, anti-inflammatory, immunoregulatory, and growth-promoting properties, which contribute to prevention of BT in VLBW infants.[50,57,65,78–94] Recombinant human LF was studied in preclinical models for its ability to prevent NEC. Feeding of recombinant human LF to neonatal rats before inducing an intestinal infection with enteroinvasive E coli was shown to enhance survival of the rat pups, reduce infection of the jejunum and ileum,[80] and limit E coli–related translocation to the liver and blood.[81] These studies were the basis for a clinical trial of bovine LF (bLF) prophylaxis in VLBW infants. Manzoni and colleagues[82] observed a significant reduction in LOS among VLBW infants fed bLF. When bLF and Lactobacillus rhamnosus GG were given enterally to the infants, NEC was significantly lower compared with controls. No adverse events were seen related to feeding bLF to infants.

Probiotic Bacteria and Prevention of Bacterial Translocation in Infants

In 1907, Nobel laureate Elie Metchnikoff proposed that yogurt (containing probiotics) prolonged life.[95] In 1899, his colleague at the Pasteur Institute, pediatrician Henry Tissier, had already discovered bifidobacteria in the feces of breastfed infants.[95]

Table 2 Mechanisms by which LF prevents gram-positive and gram-negative bacterial translocation		
Physiologic or Immune Processes Related to LF or Its Enzymatic Digestion Products	**Type of Action**	**References**
Fe^{3+} withholding defense mediates bacteriostasis	Antimicrobial	51,78,79
Synergy with peptide antibiotics (eg, lysozyme), antibiotic drugs, IgA to facilitate microbial killing	Antimicrobial	83
Low pH and peptic digest of LF kills gram-positive and gram-negative bacteria, fungi, viruses, and parasites	Antimicrobial	51,78,79
LF-derived peptides kill antibiotic-resistant *Staphylococcus aureus* and *E coli*	Antimicrobial	84,85
Binds endotoxins, exotoxins, CpG, flagellin; blocks toxin-mediated cytokine production	Anti-inflammatory	79,86–88
Blocks adhesins on cells for bacteria and biofilms Inhibits type III secretory system, flagella motility	Antimicrobial anti-inflammatory	89
Multiple enzyme activities (eg, ribonuclease)	Antimicrobial	50,57,78,90
Binds to and promotes growth of probiotic bacteria	Antimicrobial	91
Binds to intelectin, promotes proliferation and differentiation of epithelia and immune cells; primes Th1 immunity (Th2 to Th1 switch)	Antimicrobial Immunoregulatory	72,78,79,92
Activates macrophages via TLR, other receptors Recruits and activates macrophages, dendritic cells	Proinflammatory, alarmin	93,94

The bifidogenic effect of human milk is attributed to its low protein content as well as its lactose, nucleotides, oligosaccharides, and LF.[96] There is evidence that emergence of lactic acid bacteria and bifidobacteria in the nascent bowel microbiota hinders BT into the intestinal wall. *Streptococcus thermophilus* and *Lactobacillus acidophilus* interact directly with intestinal epithelia to resist *E coli*–related invasion.[97] Bioactive factors secreted by *B infantis* lessen intestinal permeability caused by TNF-α and interferon-γ.[98] Prophylaxis with *Lactobacillus plantarum* likewise prevents changes in tight junction proteins during gut-related infection with enteroinvasive *E coli*.[99] Cytokine-induced apoptosis of gut epithelia is mitigated by *Lactobacillus rhamnosus* GG.[100] Preclinical studies showed that bifidobacteria significantly moderates NEC in neonatal rats.[101]

Beneficial in vivo effects of oral probiotic biotherapy in neonates are reportedly related to more competent gut-related immunity, a less pathogenic intestinal microflora, and diminished intraluminal microbial toxins.[5,101,102] Clinical studies in human newborn infants demonstrated that probiotics reduced the incidence of NEC, although the effect was less evident in extremely preterm infants.[103,104] From a safety perspective, no probiotic bacteria were isolated from blood cultures. Probiotics have not been shown to reduce mortality, however. A meta-analysis of all probiotic studies to prevent NEC reached similar conclusions.[105] More studies with probiotics are needed to show efficacy and safety.[106]

Prebiotics and Prevention of Bacterial Translocation in Infants

When taken orally, prebiotics are nondigestible foods that selectively promote growth of one or more bacteria living in the GI tract.[107] Prebiotics in human milk include oligosaccharides and other glycans, such as glycoproteins, glycolipids, glycoaminoglycans, and mucins.[108] These milk components promote gut colonization with bifidobacteria. Some researchers suggest that the bifidogenic effect of human milk extends beyond glycans.[96] Among many bifidobacteria tested, only *Bifidobacterium longum* biovar *infantis* was able to grow during human milk oligosaccharide supplementation alone.[109] There seems to be coevolution of human milk oligosaccharides and bifidobacteria. This finding has guided research toward examining the genetic relationship of milk oligosaccharides in a mother and the emergence of her infant's intestinal microbiota.[109] In addition to the health benefits afforded by bifidobacteria, glycans may (1) inhibit bacterial and viral pathogens from binding to intestinal epithelia, (2) detoxify intraluminal products released by pathogens, (3) dampen inflammation initiated by pathogens, and (4) assist in development of innate immunity in the gut.[108,110] VLBW infants receiving a mixture of neutral and acidic oligosaccharides, however, have not exhibited a significant reduction in serious infectious morbidity.[111] Research by German and colleagues[109] has shown that oligosaccharides in mother's milk confer advantages unique to her infant, whereas formula supplemented with oligosaccharides cannot replicate the effect of mother's-own milk. A worrisome report found newborn rats fed galacto-oligosaccharides and inulin had increased bacterial translocation.[112] No studies have examined the effect of prebiotics alone on the incidence of NEC.[113] Probiotic and prebiotic mixtures are fed because they foster development of a gut-related bifidus flora akin to that in breastfed infants.[114] If a combined probiotic and prebiotic strategy is used to prevent NEC in VLBW newborns, the risk of BT necessitates frequent assessments of morbidity.

SUMMARY

Bacterial translocation from the GI tract is an important pathway initiating late-onset sepsis and necrotizing enterocolitis in very low-birth-weight infants. The emerging intestinal microbiota, nascent intestinal epithelia, naive immunity, and suboptimal nutrition (lack of breast milk) have roles in facilitating bacterial translocation. Feeding lactoferrin, probiotics, or prebiotics has presented exciting possibilities to prevent bacterial translocation in preterm infants, and clinical trials will identify the most safe and efficacious prevention and treatment strategies.

REFERENCES

1. Stoll BJ, Hansen N, Fanaroff AA, et al. Late-onset sepsis in very low birth weight neonates: the experience of the NICHD Neonatal Research Network. Pediatrics 2002;110(2):285–91.
2. Stoll BJ, Hansen NI, Adams-Chapman I, et al. Neurodevelopmental and growth impairment among extremely low-birth-weight infants with neonatal infection. JAMA 2004;292(19):2357–65.
3. Berg RD, Garlington AW. Translocation of certain indigenous bacteria from the gastrointestinal tract to the mesenteric lymph nodes and other organs in gnotobiotic mouse model. Infect Immun 1979;23(2):403–11.
4. Gatt M, Reddy BS, MacFie J. Review article: bacterial translocation in the critically ill—evidence and methods of prevention. Aliment Pharmacol Ther 2007; 25(7):741–57.

5. Hunter CJ, Upperman JS, Ford HR, et al. Understanding the susceptibility of the premature infant to necrotizing enterocolitis (NEC). Pediatr Res 2008;63(2):117–23.
6. Sharma R, Tepas JJ 3rd, Hudak ML, et al. Neonatal gut barrier and multiple organ failure: role of endotoxins and proinflammatory cytokines in sepsis and necrotizing enterocolitis. J Pediatr Surg 2007;42(3):454–61.
7. Duffy LC. Symposium: bioactivity in milk and bacterial interactions in the developing immature intestine. J Nutr 2000;130(Suppl 2S):432S–6S.
8. Hooper LV, Wong MH, Thelin A, et al. Molecular analysis of commensal host-microbial relationships in the intestine. Science 2001;291(5505):881–4.
9. Rønnestad A, Abrahamsen TG, Medbø S, et al. Late-onset septicemia in a Norwegian national cohort of extremely premature infants receiving early full human milk feeding. Pediatrics 2005;115(3):e269–76.
10. Adlerberth I, Lindberg E, Åberg N, et al. Reduced enterobacterial and increased staphylococcal colonization of the infantile bowel: an effect of hygienic lifestyle? Pediatr Res 2005;59(1):96–101.
11. Westerbeek EA, van den Berg A, Lafeber HN, et al. The intestinal bacterial colonization in preterm infants: a review of the literature. Clin Nutr 2006;25(3):361–8.
12. Neu J, Mshvildadze M, Mai V. A roadmap for understanding and preventing necrotizing enterocolitis. Curr Gastroenterol Rep 2008;10(5):450–7.
13. Björkström MV, Hall L, Söderlund S, et al. Intestinal flora in very-low birth weight infants. Acta Paediatr 2009;98(11):1762–7.
14. Hill HR, Hunt CE, Matsen JM. Nosocomial colonization with Klebsiella, type 26, in a neonatal intensive-care unit associated with an outbreak of sepsis, meningitis, and necrotizing enterocolitis. J Pediatr 1974;85(3):415–9.
15. Scheifele DW, Bjornson GL, Dyer RA, et al. Delta-like toxin produced by coagulase-negative staphylococci is associated with neonatal necrotizing enterocolitis. Infect Immun 1987;55(9):2268–73.
16. Overturf GD, Sherman MP, Scheifele DW, et al. Neonatal necrotizing enterocolitis associated with delta-toxin producing methicillin-resistant Staphylococcus aureus. Pediatr Infect Dis J 1990;9(2):88–91.
17. Frank DN, Pace NR. Gastrointestinal microbiology enters the metagenomics era. Curr Opin Gastroenterol 2008;24(1):4–10.
18. Brugère JF, Mihajlovski A, Missaoui M, et al. Tools for stools: the challenge of assessing human intestinal microbiota using molecular diagnostics. Expert Rev Mol Diagn 2009;9(4):353–65.
19. Morowitz MJ, Poroyko V, Caplan M, et al. Redefining the role of intestinal microbes in the pathogenesis of necrotizing enterocolitis. Pediatrics 2010; 125(4):777–85.
20. de la Cochetiere MF, Piloquet H, des Robert C, et al. Early intestinal bacterial colonization and necrotizing enterocolitis in premature infants: the putative role of Clostridium. Pediatr Res 2004;56(3):366–70.
21. Wang Y, Hoenig JD, Malin KJ, et al. 16S rRNA gene-based analysis of fecal microbiota from preterm infants with and without necrotizing enterocolitis. ISME J 2009;3(8):944–54.
22. Mshvildadze M, Neu J, Shuster J, et al. Intestinal microbial ecology in premature infants assessed with non-culture-based techniques. J Pediatr 2010;156(2):20–5.
23. Baker PI, Love DR, Ferguson LR. Role of gut microbiota in Crohn's disease. Expert Rev Gastroenterol Hepatol 2009;3(5):535–46.
24. Phalipon A, Sansonetti PJ. Shigellosis: innate mechanisms of inflammatory destruction of intestinal epithelium, adaptive immune response, and vaccine development. Crit Rev Immunol 2003;23(5–6):371–401.

25. Turnbaugh PJ, Ley RE, Hamady M, et al. The human microbiome project. Nature 2007;449(7164):804–10.
26. Burns JL, Griffith A, Barry JJ, et al. Transcytosis of gastrointestinal epithelial cells by Escherichia coli K1. Pediatr Res 2001;49(1):30–7.
27. Lu L, Walker WA. Pathologic and physiologic interactions of bacteria with the gastrointestinal epithelium. Am J Clin Nutr 2001;73(Suppl):1124S–30S.
28. Stebbins CE. Structural microbiology at the pathogen–host interface. Cell Microbiol 2005;7(9):1227–36.
29. Cossart P, Sansonetti PJ. Bacterial invasion: the paradigms of enteroinvasive pathogens. Science 2004;304(5668):242–8.
30. Luck SN, Bennett-Wood V, Poon R, et al. Invasion of epithelial cells by locus of enterocytes effacement-negative enterohemorrhagic Escherichia coli. Infect Immun 2005;73(5):3063–71.
31. Berin MC, Dareuille-Michaud A, Egan LJ, et al. Role of EHEC O157:H7 virulence factors in the activation of intestinal epithelial cell NF-kB and MAP kinase pathways and the upregulated expression of interleukin 8. Cell Immunol 2002;4(10):635–47.
32. Ruchaud-Sparagano MH, Maresca M, Kenny B. Enteropathogenic Escherichia coli (EPEC) inactivate innate immune responses prior to compromising epithelial barrier function. Cell Immunol 2007;9(8):1909–21.
33. Anand RJ, Leaphart CL, Mollen KP, et al. The role of the intestinal barrier in the pathogenesis of necrotizing enterocolitis. Shock 2007;27(2):124–33.
34. Kim KP, Loessner MJ. Enterobacter sakazakii invasion in human intestinal Caco-2 cells requires the host cell cytoskeleton and is enhanced by disruption of tight junctions. Infect Immun 2008;76(2):562–70.
35. Friedemann M. Epidemiology of invasive neonatal Cronobacter (Enterobacter sakazakii) infections. Eur J Clin Microbiol Infect Dis 2009;28(11):1297–304.
36. Neal MD, Leaphart C, Levy R, et al. Enterocyte TLR4 mediates phagocytosis and translocation of bacteria across the intestinal barrier. J Immunol 2006; 176(5):3070–9.
37. Kalischuk LD, Inglis GD, Buret AG. Campylobacter jejuni induces transcellular translocation of commensal bacteria via lipid rafts. Gut Pathog 2009;1(1):2.
38. Weber B, Saurer L, Mueller C. Intestinal macrophages: differentiation and involvement in intestinal immunopathologies. Semin Immunopathol 2009;31(2):171–84.
39. Van der Zanden EP, Snoek SA, Heinsbroek SE, et al. Vagus nerve activity augments intestinal macrophage phagocytosis via nicotinic acetylcholine receptor alpha4beta2. Gastroenterology 2009;137(3):1029–39 1039.e1–4.
40. Kessler W, Traeger T, Westerholt A, et al. The vagal nerve as a link between the nervous and immune system in the instance of polymicrobial sepsis. Langenbecks Arch Surg 2006;391(2):83–7.
41. Tracey KJ. Physiology and immunology of the cholinergic antiinflammatory pathway. J Clin Invest 2007;117(2):289–96.
42. Van der Zanden EP, Boeckxstaens GE, de Jonge WJ. The vagus nerve as a modulator of intestinal inflammation. Neurogastroenterol Motil 2009;21(1):6–17.
43. Caprilli R, Frieri G. The dyspeptic macrophage 30 years later: an update in the pathogenesis of Crohn's disease. Dig Liver Dis 2009;41(2):166–8.
44. Sansonetti PJ, Phalipon A. M cells as ports of entry for enteroinvasive pathogens: mechanisms of interaction, consequences for the disease process. Semin Immunol 1999;11(3):192–203.
45. Kadaoui KA, Corthésy B. Secretory IgA mediates bacterial translocation to dendritic cells in mouse Peyer's patches with restriction to mucosal compartment. J Immunol 2007;179(11):7751–7.

46. McGuckin MA, Eri R, Simms LA, et al. Intestinal barrier dysfunction in inflammatory bowel diseases. Inflamm Bowel Dis 2009;15(1):100–13.
47. Snoeck V, Goddeerie B, Cox E. The role of enterocytes in the intestinal barrier function and antigen uptake. Microbes Infect 2005;7(7–8):997–1004.
48. O'Neil DA, Porter EM, Elewaut D, et al. Expression and regulation of the human β-defensins hBD-1 and hBD-2 in intestinal epithelium. J Immunol 1999;163(12):6718–24.
49. Hase K, Eckmann L, Leopard JD, et al. Cell differentiation is a key determinant of cathelicidin LL-37/human cationic antimicrobial protein 18 expression by human colonic epithelium. Infect Immun 2002;70(2):953–63.
50. Salzman NH, Underwood MA, Bevins CL. Paneth cells, defensins, and the commensal microbiota: a hypothesis on intimate interplay at the intestinal mucosa. Semin Immunol 2007;19(2):70–83.
51. Mukherjee S, Vaishnava S, Hooper LV. Multi-layered regulation of intestinal antimicrobial defense. Cell Mol Life Sci 2008;65(19):3019–27.
52. Hooper LV, Stappenbeck TS, Hong CV, et al. Angiogenins: a new class of microbicidal proteins involved in innate immunity. Nat Immunol 2003;4(3):269–73.
53. Eckmann L. Innate immunity and mucosal bacterial interactions in the intestine. Curr Opin Gastroenterol 2004;20(2):82–8.
54. Schaart MW, de Bruijn AC, Sclerbeek H, et al. Small intestinal MUC2 synthesis in human preterm infants. Am J Physiol Gastrointest Liver Physiol 2009;296(5): G1085–90.
55. Chambers JA, Hollingsworth MA, Trezise AE, et al. Developmental expression of mucin genes MUC1 and MUC2. J Cell Sci 1994;107(Pt 2):413–24.
56. Kosloske AM, Musemeche CA. Necrotizing enterocolitis of the neonate. Clin Perinatol 1989;16(1):97–111.
57. Stappenbeck TS, Hooper LV, Gordon JI. Developmental regulation of intestinal angiogenesis by indigenous microbes via Paneth cells. Proc Natl Acad Sci U S A 2002;99(24):15451–5.
58. Mallow EB, Harris A, Salzman N, et al. Human enteric defensins. Gene structure and developmental expression. J Biol Chem 1996;2719(8):4038–45.
59. Salzman NH, Polin RA, Harris MC, et al. Enteric defensin expression in necrotizing enterocolitis. Pediatr Res 1998;44(1):20–6.
60. Coutinho HB, da Mota HC, Coutinho VB, et al. Absence of lysozyme (muramidase) in the intestinal Paneth cells of newborn infants with necrotising enterocolitis. J Clin Pathol 1998;51(7):512–4.
61. Sherman MP, Bennett SH, Hwang FF, et al. Paneth cells and antibacterial host defense in neonatal small intestine. Infect Immun 2005;73(9):6143–6.
62. Salzman NH, Hung K, Haribhai D, et al. Enteric defensins are essential regulators of intestinal microbial ecology. Nat Immunol 2010;11(1):76–83.
63. Wehkamp J, Harder J, Weichenthal M, et al. NOD2 (CARD15) mutations in Crohn's disease are associated with diminished mucosal α-defensin expression. Gut 2004;53(11):1658–64.
64. Dinsdale D, Biles B. Postnatal changes in the distribution and elemental composition of Paneth cells in normal and corticosteroid-treated rats. Cell Tissue Res 1986;246(1):183–7.
65. Halac E, Halac J, Bégué EF, et al. Prenatal and postnatal corticosteroid therapy to prevent neonatal necrotizing enterocolitis, a controlled trial. J Pediatr 1990; 117(1 Pt 1):132–8.
66. Vaishnava S, Behrendt C, Ismail AS, et al. Paneth cells directly sense gut commensals and maintain homeostasis at the intestinal host–microbial interface. Proc Natl Acad Sci U S A 2008;105(52):20858–63.

67. Tan X, Hsueh W, Gonzalez-Crussi F. Cellular localization of tumor necrosis factor (TNF)-α transcripts in normal bowel and in necrotizing enterocolitis. Am J Pathol 1993;142(6):1858–65.
68. Steenwinckel V, Louahed J, Lemaire MM, et al. IL-9 promotes IL-13-dependent Paneth cell hyperplasia and up-regulation of innate immunity mediators in intestinal mucosa. J Immunol 2009;182(8):4737–43.
69. Underwood MA, Gilbert WM, Sherman MP. Amniotic fluid: not just fetal urine anymore. J Perinatol 2005;25(5):341–8.
70. Wagner CL, Taylor SN, Johnson D. Host factors in amniotic fluid and breast milk that contribute to gut maturation. Clin Rev Allergy Immunol 2008;34(2):191–204.
71. Tunzi CR, Harper PA, Bar-Oz B, et al. Beta-defensin expression in human mammary gland epithelia. Pediatr Res 2000;48(1):30–5.
72. Takahata Y, Takada H, Nomura A, et al. Interleukin-18 in human milk. Pediatr Res 2001;50(2):268–72.
73. Vidal K, Donnel-Hughes A. CD14: a soluble pattern recognition receptor in milk. Adv Exp Med Biol 2008;606:195–216.
74. Martin R, Langa S, Reviriego C, et al. Human milk is a source of lactic acid bacteria for the infant gut. J Pediatr 2003;143(6):754–8.
75. Martin R, Jiménez E, Heilig H, et al. Isolation of bifidobacteria from breast milk and assessment of the bifidobacterial population by PCR-denaturing gradient gel electrophoresis and quantitative real-time PCR. Appl Environ Microbiol 2009;75(4):965–9.
76. Brandtzaeg P. The mucosal immune system and its integration with the mammary glands. J Pediatr 2010;156(2):S8–15.
77. Sullivan S, Schanler RJ, Kim JH, et al. An exclusively human milk-based diet is associated with a lower rate of necrotizing enterocolitis than a diet of human milk and bovine milk-based products. J Pediatr 2010;156(4):562–7, e1.
78. González-Chávez SA, Arévalo-Gallegos S, Rascón-Cruz Q. Lactoferrin: structure, function, and applications. Int J Antimicrob Agents 2009;33(4):301, e1–8.
79. Legrand D, Mazurier J. A critical review of the roles of host lactoferrin in immunity. Biometals 2010;23(3):365–76.
80. Sherman MP, Bennett SH, Hwang FF, et al. Neonatal small bowel epithelia: enhancing anti-bacterial defense with lactoferrin and Lactobacillus GG. Biometals 2004;17(3):285–9.
81. Edde L, Hipolito RB, Hwang FF, et al. Lactoferrin protects neonatal rats from gut-related systemic infection. Am J Physiol Gastrointest Liver Physiol 2001;281(5):1140–50.
82. Manzoni P, Rinaldi M, Cattani S, et al. Bovine lactoferrin supplementation for prevention of late-onset sepsis in very low-birth-weight neonates: a randomized trial. JAMA 2009;302(13):1421–8.
83. Singh PK, Tack BF, McCray PB Jr, et al. Synergistic and additive killing by antimicrobial factors found in human airway surface liquid. Am J Physiol Lung Cell Mol Physiol 2000;279(5):L799–805.
84. Haney EF, Nazmi K, Lau F, et al. Novel lactoferrampin antimicrobial peptides derived from human lactoferrin. Biochimie 2009;91(1):141–54.
85. Flores-Villaseñor H, Canizalez-Román A, Reyes-Lopez M, et al. Bactericidal effect of bovine lactoferrin, LFcin, LFampin, and LFchimera on antibiotic-resistant *Staphylococcus aureus* and *Escherichia coli*. Biometals 2010;23(3):569–78.
86. Baveye S, Elass E, Fernig DG, et al. Human lactoferrin interacts with soluble CD14 and inhibits expression of endothelial adhesion molecules, E-selectin,

        and ICAM-1, induced by the CD14-lipopolysachharide complex. Infect Immun
        2000;68(12):6519–25.
87. Mulligan P, White NR, Monteleone G, et al. Breast milk lactoferrin regulates gene
     expression by binding bacterial DNA CpG motifs but not genomic DNA
     promoters in model intestinal cells. Pediatr Res 2006;59(5):656–61.
88. Hayworth JL, Kasper KJ, Leon-Ponte M, et al. Attenuation of massive cyto-
     kine response to the staphylococcal enterotoxin B superantigen by the
     innate immunomodulatory protein lactoferrin. Clin Exp Immunol 2009;
     157(1):60–70.
89. Ochoa TJ, Cleary TG. Effect of lactoferrin on enteric pathogens. Biochimie 2009;
     91(1):30–4.
90. Kanyshkova TG, Babina SE, Semenov DV, et al. Multiple enzymatic activities of
     human milk lactoferrin. Eur J Biochem 2003;270(16):3353–61.
91. Rahman MM, Kim WS, Ito T, et al. Growth promotion and cell binding ability of
     bovine lactoferrin to Bifidobacterium longum. Anaerobe 2009;15(4):133–7.
92. Legrand D, Elass E, Carpentier M, et al. Interactions of lactoferrin with cells
     involved with immune function. Biochem Cell Biol 2006;84(3):282–90.
93. Curren CS, Demick KP, Mansfield JM. Lactoferrin activates macrophages via
     TLR4-dependent and -independent signaling pathways. Cell Immunol 2006;
     242(1):23–30.
94. Yang D, de la Rosa G, Tewary P, et al. Alarmins link neutrophils and dendritic
     cells. Trends Immunol 2009;30(11):531–7.
95. Shortt C. The probiotic century: historical and current perspectives. Trends Food
     Sci Technol 1999;10:411–7.
96. Coppa GV, Zampini L, Galeazzi T, et al. Prebiotics in human milk: a review. Dig
     Liver Dis 2006;38(Suppl 2):S291–4.
97. Resta-Lenert S, Barrett KE. Live probiotics protect intestinal epithelial cells from
     the effects of infection with enteroinvasive Escherichia coli (EIEC). Gut 2003;
     52(7):988–97.
98. Ewaschuk JB, Diaz H, Meddings L, et al. Secreted bioactive factors from Bifido-
     bacterium infantis enhance epithelial barrier function. Am J Physiol Gastrointest
     Liver Physiol 2008;295(5):G1025–34.
99. Qin H, Zhang Z, Hang X, et al. L. plantarum prevents enteroinvasive Escherichia
     coli-induced tight junction proteins changes in intestinal epithelial cells. BMC
     Microbiol 2009;31(9):63.
100. Yan F, Polk DB. Probiotic bacterium prevents cytokine-induced apoptosis in
     intestinal epithelial cells. J Biol Chem 2002;277(52):50959–65.
101. Caplan MS, Miller-Catchpole R, Kaup S, et al. Bifidobacterial supplementation
     reduces the incidence of necrotizing enterocolitis in a neonatal rat model.
     Gastroenterology 1999;117(3):577–83.
102. Urao M, Fujimoto T, Lane GJ, et al. Does probiotics administration decrease
     serum endotoxins levels in infants? J Pediatr Surg 1999;34(2):273–6.
103. Bin-Nun A, Bromiker R, Wilschanski M, et al. Oral probiotics prevent necrotizing
     enterocolitis in very low birth weight neonates. J Pediatr 2005;147(2):192–6.
104. Lin HC, Hsu CH, Chen HL, et al. Oral probiotics prevent necrotizing enterocolitis
     in very low birth weight preterm infants: a multicenter, randomized, controlled
     trial. Pediatrics 2008;122(4):693–700.
105. Alfaleh K, Anabrees J, Bassler D. Probiotics reduce the risk of necrotizing
     enterocolitis in preterm infants: a meta-analysis. Neonatology 2010;97(2):93–9.
106. Liong MT. Safety of probiotics: translocation and infection. Nutr Rev 2008;66(4):
     192–202.

107. Schrezenmeir J, de Vrese M. Probiotics, prebiotics, and synbiotics—approaching a definition. Am J Clin Nutr 2001;73(Suppl):361S–4S.
108. Newburg DS. Neonatal protection by an innate immune system of human milk consisting of oligosaccharides and glycans. J Anim Sci 2009;87(Suppl 13): 27–34.
109. German JB, Freeman SL, Lebrilla CB, et al. Human milk oligosaccharides: evolution, structures and bioselectivity as substrates for intestinal bacteria. Nestle Nutr Workshop Ser Pediatr Program 2008;62:205–18 [discussion: 218–22].
110. Boehm G, Moro G. Structural and functional aspects of prebiotics used in infant nutrition. J Nutr 2008;138(9):1818S–28S.
111. Westerbeek EA, van den Berg JP, Lafeber HN, et al. Neutral and acidic oligosaccharides in preterm infants: a randomized, double-blind, placebo-controlled trial. Am J Clin Nutr 2010;91(3):679–86.
112. Barrat E, Michel C, Poupeau G, et al. Supplementation with galactooligosaccharides and inulin increases bacterial translocation in artificially reared newborn rats. Pediatr Res 2008;64(1):34–9.
113. Caplan MS. Probiotic and prebiotic supplementation for the prevention of neonatal necrotizing enterocolitis. J Perinatol 2009;29(Suppl 2):S2–6.
114. Bakker-Zierikee AM, Alles MS, Knol J, et al. Effects of infant formula containing a mixture of galacto- and fructo-oligosaccharides or viable *Bifidobacterium animalis* on the intestinal microflora during the first 4 months of life. Br J Nutr 2005; 94(5):783–90.

Heart Rate Characteristics: Physiomarkers for Detection of Late-Onset Neonatal Sepsis

Karen D. Fairchild, MD[a],*, T. Michael O'Shea, MD[b]

KEYWORDS

• Heart rate variability • Heart rate characteristics
• Neonatal sepsis • Cytokines

TOWARD AN EARLIER DIAGNOSIS OF LATE-ONSET NEONATAL SEPSIS IN PATIENTS IN THE NEONATAL INTENSIVE CARE UNIT

Late-onset neonatal sepsis (LONS) kills thousands of preterm infants in the United States each year, and many survivors develop permanent neurologic impairment.[1,2] Typically, after a patient in the neonatal intensive care unit (NICU) develops signs and symptoms of sepsis, tests are sent and antibiotic therapy and other supportive care is initiated. However, waiting for a baby to deteriorate clinically is suboptimal and results in mortality rates as high as 40%. Earlier detection and treatment of LONS offers the best opportunity to improve outcomes. To date, the approach has been to use biomarker screening or empiric antibiotic therapy for every patient with subtle nonspecific symptoms. Neither of these strategies is satisfactory because of the insufficient diagnostic accuracy of biomarkers and complications associated with overuse of antibiotics. A new technology, continuous monitoring of neonatal heart rate characteristics (HRC), has been developed for the earlier diagnosis and treatment of LONS in patients in the NICU.[3–9] This article reviews the physiology of heart rate variability (HRV) in healthy and diseased states, with particular focus on the role of

Funding sources: NIH HD048562 (J.R. Moorman, PI), NIH HD051609 (K.D.F.), Coulter Foundation Translational Research Award, and University of Virginia Children's Hospital Grants.
[a] Division of Neonatology, University of Virginia, Hospital Drive, Charlottesville, VA 22908, USA
[b] Division of Neonatology, Wake Forest University, Medical Center Boulevard, Winston-Salem, NC 27104, USA
* Corresponding author.
E-mail address: kdf2n@virginia.edu

Clin Perinatol 37 (2010) 581–598
doi:10.1016/j.clp.2010.06.002
0095-5108/10/$ – see front matter © 2010 Elsevier Inc. All rights reserved.

perinatology.theclinics.com

the autonomic nervous system and inflammation in decreased HRV in sepsis. The authors also review research showing that continuous monitoring of HRC in patients in the NICU can detect LONS often in its early stages before the onset of symptoms. A randomized clinical trial to assess the effect of continuous HRC monitoring in 3000 preterm infants will be complete in 2010, and it is important for clinicians to understand the basis of this new technology.

HRV AND HRC

In healthy animals and humans the interval between heartbeats is not constant, but rather constantly changing. Beat-to-beat variability is regulated by neural input to the heart, with sympathetic and parasympathetic branches of the autonomic nervous system contributing to accelerations and decelerations of heart rate, respectively.[10] Heart rate and HRV are linked to other vital signs, such as respiration, temperature, and blood pressure, through reflex feedback from the central nervous system to cardiac pacemaker cells. Abnormal heart rate characteristics (HRC) in the context of neonatal sepsis detection are composed of 2 components: depressed HRV and transient heart rate decelerations. HRC analysis is described in more detail in the section on clinical research and applications of HRC monitoring in neonates, whereas the term HRV is used in the discussions of physiology of heart rate control in healthy and diseased conditions.

AUTONOMIC NERVOUS SYSTEM REGULATION OF HRV

Chronotropic regulation of the heart occurs primarily through autonomic innervation of sinoatrial (SA) node pacemaker cells. The SA node is a small region of specialized impulse-generating cells on the posterolateral wall of the right atrium at the juncture with the superior vena cava. Although other cardiomyocytes have pacemaker potential, SA node cells have a faster pacing rate and thus their signals override the intrinsic rate of other atrial and ventricular cells. The SA node is innervated by efferent autonomic nerves that release neurotransmitters and trigger changes in ion flux, resulting in heart rate accelerations and decelerations.[11]

Sympathetic Nervous System

The sympathetic nervous system (SNS) is responsible for the acute stress "fight-or-flight" response, which includes increase in heart rate and cardiac contractility and inhibition of other visceral functions, mediated in large part by the adrenomedullary release of epinephrine. Under basal conditions, the SNS also plays a role in the maintenance of physiologic homeostasis in many organ systems, including the immune system. Sympathetic sensory neurons send afferent signals to paravertebral ganglia anterior to the thoracic segment of the spinal cord. From there, postganglionic sympathetic neurons extend to the brainstem and then to the heart, lungs, and viscera, where they regulate functions through the release of norepinephrine.

The SNS plays a major role in regulating heart rate, cardiac output, peripheral vascular resistance, and blood pressure. Afferent signals arise from baroreceptors and chemoreceptors in the brainstem (medulla oblongata), carotid arteries, and aortic arch. Baroreceptors sense increases and decreases in blood pressure, and trigger sympathetic and parasympathetic responses in blood pressure and heart rate to restore homeostasis. Chemoreceptors sense changes in the concentration of carbon dioxide, oxygen, and hydrogen ion in the blood, leading to signals sent via sympathetic nerves to the diaphragm and the heart. These receptors are primarily involved in the control of breathing but can also respond to a decrease in blood pressure, causing decreased oxygen delivery to the receptors. Sympathetic nerve endings in the SA node of the heart release norepinephrine, which binds to β_1-adrenergic receptors leading to adenylyl cyclase activation, increased cyclic adenosine monophosphate, altered ion flux, faster depolarization, and increased heart rate and contractility.

Parasympathetic Nervous System

The parasympathetic nervous system (PNS) plays a critical role in regulation of heart rate and numerous other vital functions. The vagus nerve (cranial nerve X) both senses and signals physiologic changes in healthy and diseased states. In the heart, parasympathetic vagal nerve endings release acetylcholine, which binds to muscarinic cholinergic receptors on pacemaker cells, causing opening of potassium channels, hyperpolarization of the membrane, and decrease in heart rate.

Vagal Fibers-Immune-Brain Communications

The vagus nerve, in addition to playing a major role in regulation of heart rate and gastrointestinal and lung function, is also a key modulator of the host defense against infection. A 2-way interaction exists between the immune system and the brain, with afferent and efferent signals relayed via vagal fibers. The presence of peripheral infectious or inflammatory insults is relayed to the brain by vagal afferent nerve fibers (**Fig. 1**). For example, animal models have demonstrated that intraperitoneal administration of endotoxin from gram-negative bacteria or proinflammatory cytokines such as interleukin (IL)-1β results in rapid signaling via abdominal branches of the vagus nerve to nuclei in the brainstem. Vagal motor efferent neurons then stimulate physiologic changes in the brain including fever, and "sickness behaviors" such as anorexia and apathy.[12] Effects of vagal efferent signaling on the heart during sepsis are not well studied, but could include heart rate decelerations as found in mice immediately after intraperitoneal endotoxin administration[13] and in neonates with sepsis.

The vagus nerve also serves a potent anti-inflammatory function. Tracey and colleagues[14,15] discovered that vagal efferent signaling significantly dampens the production of proinflammatory cytokines. The effect, termed the cholinergic anti-inflammatory response, results from acetylcholine binding to nicotinic acetylcholine receptors on tissue macrophages, resulting in decreased activation of the transcription factor nuclear factor κB and decreased release of tumor necrosis factor α, IL-1β, and other cytokines.[14,15] In animal models of sepsis, vagotomy increases cytokine production and mortality, whereas electrical stimulation of the vagus nerve or pharmacotherapy with nicotine or nicotinic cholinergic receptor agonists reduces cytokine production and mortality.[16,17] Recent research indicates that activation of the cholinergic anti-inflammatory pathway could also be beneficial in sepsis-associated acute lung injury[18,19] and neuroinflammation.[20]

HUMORAL AND MECHANICAL FACTORS CONTRIBUTING TO HRV

Although direct neurotransmitter release at the SA node is the major mediator of heart rate accelerations and decelerations, there is also evidence of indirect humoral and mechanical (stretch) effects on heart rate and its variability. In denervated hearts, limited variability in the beating rate has been observed. Mechanoreceptors in the atrium respond to stretch (such as that which occurs during normal respiration with changes in intrathoracic volume and venous return) and directly signal changes in heart rate without neural input.[21] Systemic release of adrenomedullary catecholamines in response to stress can lead to increased heart rate in the absence of sympathetic nerve firing to pacemaker cells. Glucocorticoids have also

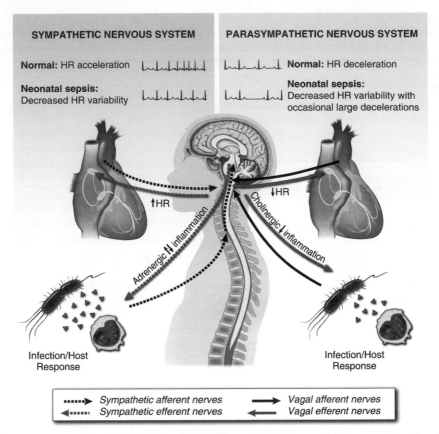

Fig. 1. Immune-nervous system-heart interactions. Pathogens or cytokines send impulses to the brainstem via afferent nerves. Afferent autonomic signals are also triggered by baroreceptors in response to changes in blood pressure. Sympathetic and parasympathetic (vagus) nerves then send efferent signals to the SA node, leading to compensatory heart rate (HR) accelerations and decelerations, respectively. In sepsis, there is decreased HRV with fewer small accelerations and decelerations, likely reflecting dysregulation of autonomic responses. Neonates with sepsis may have both decreased HRV and occasional large decelerations. The autonomic nervous system, in addition to regulating HRV, also plays an important role in host defense by sending adrenergic and cholinergic signals to the periphery modulating release of inflammatory mediators such as cytokines. (*Courtesy of* Anita Impagliazzo, MA, CMI; copyright 2010; with permission.)

been found to enhance HRV in both animals and humans. The authors' group has demonstrated that mice treated with dexamethasone experienced a 2- to 3-fold increase in various measures of HRV even in the absence of an inflammatory insult.[13] Fetal HRV is also increased acutely following maternal administration of dexamethasone or betamethasone.[22] In adults with sepsis, adrenal insufficiency is associated with depressed HRV, whereas glucocorticoid treatment leads to normalization of HRV.[23] Effects of glucocorticoids on HRV may be dose specific, as a study in healthy adults showed that continuous infusion of low-dose hydrocortisone did not alter baseline HRV or cause HRV changes in response to endotoxin administration.[24]

RELATIONSHIP BETWEEN HEART RATE, HRV, AND OTHER VITAL SIGNS

The centuries-old observation that heart rate increases during inhalation and decreases during exhalation is termed respiratory sinus arrhythmia (RSA). This normal physiologic phenomenon involves an increase in intrathoracic volume during inspiration, resulting in an increase in sympathetic tone and a decrease in parasympathetic tone, leading to increased heart rate. RSA may play a role in maintaining ventilation-perfusion matching through the 2 phases of respiration. RSA is reflected in high-frequency HRV, with accelerations occurring at 0.15 to 0.4 Hz, or 9 to 24 cycles per minute, the normal respiratory rate in adults. High-frequency HRV is widely accepted as a measure of vagal tone in adults, whereas low-frequency HRV is thought to reflect both sympathetic and parasympathetic input to the heart. Because neonates typically breathe about 3 times faster than adults, the frequency range for RSA (high-frequency HRV) is higher.

Breathing also contributes to HRV through the chemoreceptor reflex and the sympathetic arm of the autonomic nervous system. Central chemoreceptors in the brainstem and peripheral chemoreceptors in the carotid sinus and aortic arch detect levels of carbon dioxide, oxygen, and hydrogen ions in the blood and trigger action potentials, which travel along afferent nerves to sympathetic ganglia. Postganglionic sympathetic nerve fibers then extend to an effector organ such as the diaphragm (triggering inspiration) or the heart (triggering norepinephrine release and increased beating rate).

Body temperature seems to play a relatively minor role in HRV. It is well known that hypothermia is associated with sinus bradycardia, and fever with tachycardia, but the contribution of baseline heart rate to HRV seems to be small. Fluctuations in body temperature may be reflected in changes in HRV in the very low– and ultralow-frequency ranges.

Blood pressure affects heart rate through the baroreceptor reflex. In response to high blood pressure, stretch-sensitive receptors in the carotid sinus and aortic arch send action potentials via the vagus and glossopharyngeal nerves to the solitary tract nucleus (NTS) of the brainstem. The NTS in turn triggers the ventrolateral medulla to send inhibitory signals to the SNS and triggers the nucleus ambiguus to activate the PNS. The net result is decreased heart rate and decreased blood pressure. In response to hypotension, the baroreceptor reflex works in reverse, increasing sympathetic tone and decreasing vagal tone to raise the blood pressure and heart rate.

MEASUREMENT OF HRV

HRV analysis is generally performed using linear time-domain or frequency-domain methods, but can also be accomplished with nonlinear methods as reviewed elsewhere.[25]

Time-domain analysis of HRV primarily involves calculation of the standard deviation of normal R-R intervals in the electrocardiogram (ECG). Aberrant beats and artifacts are removed before analysis. Multiple other time-domain measures are also used for clinical research.[26] Frequency-domain analysis or power spectral analysis may be used to determine the relative contribution of parasympathetic neural input to HRV. ECG time-series data are transformed to quantitate variability (power) within different frequency ranges. The 2 major spectra in adult humans are high frequency, 0.15 to 0.4 Hz or 9 to 24 cycles per minute, and low frequency, 0.04 to 0.15 Hz. High-frequency fluctuations in heart rate reflect rapid vagal responses to breathing, whereas the response of SNS to physiologic changes is slower and is reflected in low-frequency HRV.

Research into the optimum methods for analyzing HRV in neonates revealed that power spectral analysis did not add additional information to time-domain analysis for detecting sepsis.[27,28] The 3 time-based measures used for calculation of the HRC index in neonates, standard deviation of R-R intervals, sample asymmetry, and sample entropy, are discussed later in this review.

Pathologic States Associated with Abnormal HRV

Obstetricians have long known that loss of fetal HRV and repetitive heart rate decelerations are ominous signs associated with asphyxia[29] or chorioamnionitis.[30,31] In adults, several cardiovascular diseases are associated with depressed HRV, including coronary artery disease, myocardial infarction, and congestive heart failure.[10] Acute brain injury has also been linked to decreased HRV in adults, children, neonates, and fetuses.[32–36] Chronic endocrine, metabolic, and renal conditions, including diabetes, hyperglycemia, hyperlipidemia, obesity, and kidney failure, may lead to autonomic dysregulation and low HRV.[37] HRV is affected by psychiatric disorders as well, notably major depression.[38] In some of these conditions, abnormal HRV seems to be linked to overactivation of the SNS and the hypothalamic-pituitary-adrenal axis.[39]

Sepsis has a strong association with decreased HRV in animal models and in humans of all ages. In a mouse model of sepsis-like illness, administration of endotoxin from gram-negative bacteria caused a dose-dependent decrease in HRV.[13] Human volunteers who are administered intravenous endotoxin also exhibit a significant decrease in HRV, concurrent with other symptoms of illness such as fever, tachypnea, tachycardia, and hypotension.[40] In adults, children, and neonates, sepsis is associated with a decrease in multiple measures of HRV, and lower HRV generally correlates with higher illness severity scores and higher mortality.[4,41,42]

Mechanisms of Decreased HRV in Sepsis

Dampening of HRV during sepsis likely reflects the impairment of normal autonomic homeostatic functions. The precise mechanisms of this phenomenon are not well understood, but there is evidence of abnormalities of both sympathetic and parasympathetic tone during sepsis. Increasing evidence points to an important role of the systemic inflammatory response (notably, inflammatory cytokines) in decreased HRV in sepsis and other disease processes.

Autonomic Dysfunction in Sepsis

Sepsis-associated sympathetic dysfunction, both overactivation and downregulation, have been described. Although the activation of the adrenergic system in sepsis is critical for initiating a physiologic response to pathogens, it can become detrimental if excessive because the overproduction of catecholamines leads to tachycardia, diastolic dysfunction, and myocardial ischemia. Noncardiac adverse effects of sympathetic overstimulation in sepsis have also been reported, including elevated pulmonary vascular resistance and pulmonary edema, hypercoagulability, intestinal ischemia, bone marrow suppression, hyperglycemia and hyperlipidemia, and stimulation of bacterial growth.[43] There is also evidence that sepsis can lead to impaired sympathetic cardiovascular responsiveness. For example, a study of adults with sepsis found that patients with shock had higher levels of circulating norepinephrine, yet they also demonstrated decreased low-frequency HRV.[44] A small study of pediatric patients with septic shock also showed decreased low-frequency HRV in the acute phase of illness.[42] Adrenergic responsiveness has been shown to be downregulated at the cellular level in sepsis,[45,46] which may contribute to depressed HRV.

Altered vagal tone may also play a role in decreased HRV in sepsis. In an experimental model of sepsis in adults, sympathetic activation by infusion of epinephrine before administration of endotoxin reduced high-frequency HRV, suggesting vagal hyporesponsiveness.[47] It is plausible that severe sepsis could induce a state of generally decreased vagal efferent firing or responsiveness, leading to fewer normal small decelerations in heart rate. On the other hand, activation of a cholinergic anti-inflammatory response in sepsis, as previously discussed, involves vagal efferent signaling that would theoretically decrease the heart rate and increase HRV. These 2 effects could explain the findings of both reduced HRV and intermittent transient HR decelerations in neonates with sepsis, as discussed later in this review.

Cytokine Link to Decreased HRV in Sepsis and Other Diseases

Increasing evidence in both animal and human studies points to an inverse correlation between HRV and proinflammatory cytokine production in sepsis and other disease processes. The authors have shown that in mice, the administration of *Escherichia coli* endotoxin induced a dose-dependent decrease in HRV, which was temporally correlated with increased levels of multiple cytokines in the serum. Suppression of cytokine production with dexamethasone resulted in resolution of abnormal HRV, while the administration of a single cytokine, tumor necrosis factor α, was sufficient to depress HRV.[13] In a study of healthy middle-aged adults, baseline vagal tone (high-frequency HRV) was found to be inversely correlated with endotoxin-stimulated production of proinflammatory cytokines.[48] Several studies in septic adults have found an association between low HRV and high levels of cytokines.[49,50] The association between cytokines (eg, IL-6) and decreased HRV has also been made in chronic disease processes, including cardiovascular and kidney disease,[38,47,51] and in healthy adults.[52] It remains to be determined whether cytokines directly affect SA node firing or indirectly influence HRV via effects on sympathovagal function. At the in vitro level, cytokines and endotoxin have been shown to affect cardiomyocyte adrenergic receptor and ion channel functions.[53]

To summarize, experimental data from animals and observational studies in adult humans indicate that abnormal HRV is a physiomarker for processes triggered by sepsis. The authors now discuss how this physiomarker might be used as an early signal for impending sepsis in neonates.

CLINICAL RESEARCH AND APPLICATIONS OF HRC MONITORING IN NEONATES
Abnormal HRC Before Sepsis

Initial studies in the NICU tested the hypothesis that the early stages of neonatal sepsis lead to decreased HRV. These studies revealed that there was not only decreased HRV but also transient repetitive heart rate decelerations coinciding with or preceding clinical signs of sepsis. **Fig. 2** depicts both these findings at the onset of sepsis in a preterm neonate. Such abnormalities have been observed during fetal distress and severe neonatal illness.[54,55] Heart rate decelerations have not been reported in older patients with sepsis, and their cause is not well understood at present. Although some of these events could reflect breathing pauses, other mechanisms seem to be involved because the decelerations occur in patients on mechanical ventilation without a decrease in oxygen saturation. One possible explanation is intermittent vagal firing in the setting of a systemic inflammatory response.

From a practical standpoint, to detect the abnormal HRC discussed here, no additional monitoring leads are required; the information is derived from the analog ECG voltage signal from bedside monitors. This signal is digitized and filtered, and QRS

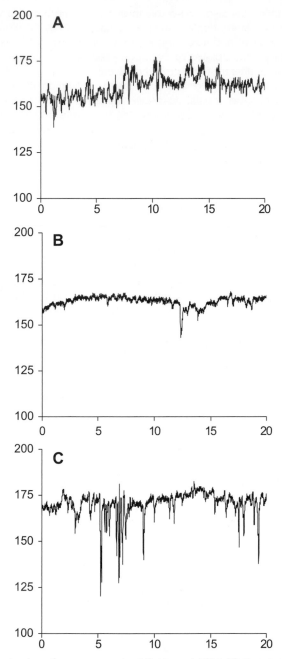

Fig. 2. Heart rate tracings from a neonate. (*A*) Normal HRV. (*B*) Decreased HRV with one deceleration. (*C*) Decreased variability with multiple superimposed transient decelerations.

complexes are identified. HRC are derived from each 4096-beat epoch of R-R intervals (approximately 20–30 minutes of ECG recording).

In an initial test of the hypothesis that sepsis is associated with both decreased HRV and decelerations, continuous monitoring was performed in 89 neonates hospitalized in the NICU at the University of Virginia.[9] Among them, 40 had one or more episodes of culture-positive sepsis (a total of 46 episodes), 23 had a total of 27 episodes of culture-negative sepsis-like illness, and 26 had neither. When compared with infants who had neither sepsis nor sepsis-like illness, infants with sepsis had reduced baseline variability and more-frequent transient decelerations. These differences were found for infants with a positive blood culture results as well as for those with culture-negative sepsis-like illness. A quantitative measure of the frequency of decelerations (ie, skewness; discussed later) began to increase as much as 24 hours before an abrupt clinical deterioration. This measure, which indirectly reports on decelerations as a tail in the histogram of R-R intervals, added to the predictive value of a validated indicator of illness severity, the Score for Neonatal Acute Physiology.[56]

HRC Index

Based on the initial clinical observations in infants with sepsis, statistical descriptors were sought to detect these abnormalities using R-R interval time series. One descriptor is the standard deviation, a conventional measure of variability. A novel measure, called sample asymmetry, detects decelerations, as indicated by asymmetry of the frequency histograms of heart rate (**Fig. 3**).[57] A symmetric histogram has a value of 1, whereas the sample asymmetry is greater than 1 for a frequency histogram with a tail to the right of the median (accelerations) and less than 1 for a frequency histogram with a tail to the left of the median (decelerations). Thus it is a more flexible and informative measure than the skewness alone.

The third mathematical measure used to detect the heart rate alterations preceding neonatal sepsis is a novel measure, prompted by the observation that approximate

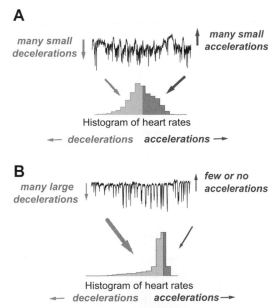

Fig. 3. Normal and abnormal heart rate histograms. (*A*) Heart rate tracing (beats per minute) from a healthy neonate showing many small heart rate accelerations and decelerations, resulting in a symmetric histogram. (*B*) Heart rate tracing from a septic neonate showing few accelerations and many large decelerations, resulting in an asymmetric histogram skewed to the left.

entropy, a measure of regularity in time-series data, is decreased in fetuses with acidosis.[55] A similar measure that was designed to have more accuracy in short records, sample entropy, decreases before clinical deterioration occurs due to sepsis.[58]

From these 3 descriptors of the R-R interval time series, an HRC index (HRCi) was developed (**Fig. 4**). HRCi is derived from the output of a logistic regression model that uses standard deviation, sample asymmetry, and sample entropy data to predict the occurrence of an acute clinical deterioration in the next 24 hours. When an individual infant's risk is divided by the average probability of a clinical deterioration (averaged over all infants and all epochs), the result is the fold increase in risk for that infant. This quantitative number is referred to as the HRCi, and is interpreted as the fold increase in risk of a clinical deterioration (clinical or culture-proven sepsis) in the next 24 hours.[8] Regression coefficients for each HRC were derived using data from 316 infants hospitalized in the years 1999 to 2001 at the University of Virginia NICU. The resulting logistic regression model was then applied to HRC data collected on 317 infants hospitalized in the years 1999 to 2001 at Wake Forest University NICU. The predictive value of the model, expressed as the area under the receiver operating characteristic (ROC) curve, was as high at the Wake Forest University NICU (the test sample) as at the University of Virginia NICU (the training sample).[7]

It is noteworthy that some patients in the NICU have multiple self-resolved increases in HRCi prior to clinical deterioration. As shown in **Fig. 5**, acute spikes in HRCi score

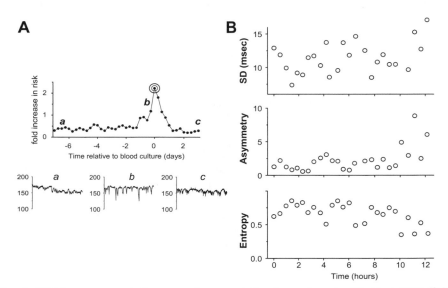

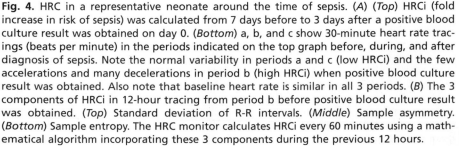

Fig. 4. HRC in a representative neonate around the time of sepsis. (*A*) (*Top*) HRCi (fold increase in risk of sepsis) was calculated from 7 days before to 3 days after a positive blood culture result was obtained on day 0. (*Bottom*) a, b, and c show 30-minute heart rate tracings (beats per minute) in the periods indicated on the top graph before, during, and after diagnosis of sepsis. Note the normal variability in periods a and c (low HRCi) and the few accelerations and many decelerations in period b (high HRCi) when positive blood culture result was obtained. Also note that baseline heart rate is similar in all 3 periods. (*B*) The 3 components of HRCi in 12-hour tracing from period b before positive blood culture result was obtained. (*Top*) Standard deviation of R-R intervals. (*Middle*) Sample asymmetry. (*Bottom*) Sample entropy. The HRC monitor calculates HRCi every 60 minutes using a mathematical algorithm incorporating these 3 components during the previous 12 hours.

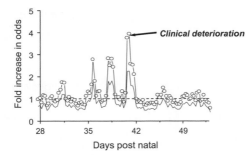

Fig. 5. Multiple spikes in HRCi before clinical deterioration with sepsis. Fold increase in odds for sepsis (HRCi) in a preterm infant aged 4 to 7 weeks. Note that the HRCi increased to approximately 2 to 3 on postnatal days 30, 36, and 39, then spontaneously returned to normal (<1). On day 41, the infant had an acute clinical deterioration associated with a positive blood culture result. When antibiotics were started, clinical status improved and the HRCi returned to normal.

may occur from the normal range (≤ 1) to more than 2-fold increase in risk of sepsis followed by spontaneous return to normal. In some cases, these self-resolved spikes are followed by acute clinical deterioration consistent with sepsis. The mechanisms and significance of this phenomenon are not precisely known. One possibility is that this phenomenon represents host defenses keeping an infection or inflammatory response under control for a time but finally breaking down, leading to clinical deterioration.

HRCi and Prediction of Sepsis

To determine the clinical utility of HRCi, data were analyzed on 678 infants admitted to the University of Virginia NICU in 1999 to 2003 and 344 infants admitted to the Wake Forest University NICU in 1999 to 2001. **Fig. 6A** illustrates the fold increased risk of an adverse event (sepsis, urinary tract infection, or death) in the next 24 hours as a function of the patient having HRCi in the high-risk range (defined as >90th percentile or score >3). HRCi in the high-risk zone was more strongly associated with sepsis than individual laboratory tests or clinical symptoms (see **Fig. 6B**).[5]

To compare the predictive value of HRCi and clinical signs of sepsis, a clinical score was developed that assigned 2 points for feeding intolerance, severe apnea, and an abnormal ratio of immature to total neutrophils (>0.2), and 1 point for increase in ventilator support, lethargy or hypotonia, temperature instability, hyperglycemia, or a white blood cell count greater than 25,000 or less than 5000.[5] The mean of this score over the entire hospital course was highly correlated with the mean HRCi, and both the clinical score and HRCi were predictive of sepsis in the next 24 hours, with the area under ROC curve being 0.62 and 0.67, respectively. The ROC curve area was 0.70 for a model containing both HRCi and clinical score, and the HRCi added significantly to the clinical score (**Fig. 7**).

Cumulative HRCi

Further validation of the significance of the HRCi was obtained from 2 studies of an index referred to as the cumulative HRCi (cHRC). cHRC was calculated as the sum, across all 6-hour epochs during an infant's NICU hospitalization, of the difference between the HRCi and the expected risk of sepsis or sepsis-like illness in the next 24 hours, based on gestational age, birth weight, and postnatal age. This cumulative

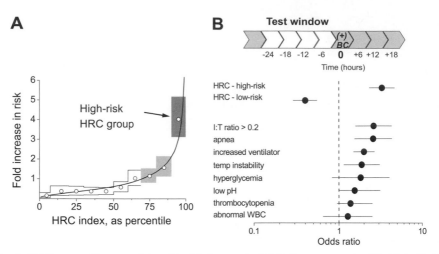

Fig. 6. HRCi percentiles correlate with risk for sepsis. (*A*) Patients were classified into 3 risk categories. Low risk is defined as HRCi less than 75th percentile (score <1). Medium risk (*light gray boxes*) includes infants with HRCi in the 75th to 90th percentile (score 1–2). The high-risk HRC group (*dark gray box*) has HRCi greater than 90th percentile (score >3). (*B*) Performance of HRCi monitoring, laboratory tests, and clinical signs for prediction of sepsis in the next 24 hours. (+) BC, positive blood culture result; I:T, immature:total neutrophils; WBC, white blood cells.

difference would be zero for the days when an infant's HRC led to a predicted risk identical to the risk predicted on the basis of gestational age, birth weight, and post-natal age. Summing this difference across all hospital days provides information as to whether the infant had a more-than-expected burden of illness (as reflected in

Heart rate characteristics

Clinical score		Not measured	Low	Inter-mediate	High
	Not measured	1.0	<1	1-2	≥2
	0	0.7	0.5	1	2.5
	1	2	1	2	4
	≥2	3	3	3	4

Fig. 7. A clinical score was developed that assigns 2 points for severe apnea, feeding intolerance, or an elevated ratio of immature to total neutrophils (>0.2), and 1 point for increase in ventilator support, lethargy or hypotonia, temperature instability, hyperglycemia, or white blood cell count more than 25,000 or less than 5000. HRC are classified as low, intermediate, or high risk for sepsis as defined in **Fig. 6**. Odds of sepsis are highest (darker gray cells) when both clinical score and HRCi are high, and lowest (white cells) when both are low. Combining HRCi monitoring with clinical risk assessment gives the best predictive accuracy for sepsis diagnosis. (*Data from* Griffin MP, Lake DE, O'Shea TM, et al. Heart rate characteristics and clinical signs in neonatal sepsis. Pediatr Res 2007;61(2):222–7.)

abnormal HRC and high cHRC) or a less-than-expected burden of illness (low cHRC). cHRC was near zero for survivors, validating the hypothesis, and was significantly higher in infants who died, suggesting that this value indicated the overall burden of disease.[59]

Furthermore, among the surviving very low birth weight (VLBW) infants, those with cerebral palsy or developmental delays (Bayley Scales of Infant Development mental or motor scores more than 2 standard deviations less than the mean) had significantly higher cHRC than infants without these developmental problems.[60]

Potential Clinical Utility of HRC Monitoring

One advantage of HRC monitoring is that it can be performed continuously and non-invasively, regardless of whether an infant is showing signs of sepsis. For the patients in the NICU whose ECG data were used to develop and validate the HRCi, the HRC data were available 92% of the time.[5] In comparison, laboratory tests used to evaluate infants for sepsis were only available a small fraction of the time. HRCi added information about the risk of sepsis over and above that provided by laboratory tests or clinical findings. An additional advantage is that HRCi often increases hours before the clinical deterioration that prompts laboratory measurements.

The research findings described earlier were based on experience with HRCi in 2 NICUs, and it remains to be determined how broadly representative these findings are. Furthermore, it is unknown whether patient outcomes are improved by HRC monitoring. This issue is being addressed by an ongoing randomized controlled trial (ClinicalTrials.gov Identifier: NCT00307333). In this study, 3000 VLBW infants are being randomized to display or no-display of the HRCi, with the primary outcome being number of days alive and not dependent on a ventilator in the 120 days after randomization. Enrollment for this trial is expected to be complete in May 2010.

The optimal strategy for using HRCi would incorporate information from both a clinical risk assessment and HRCi, an example of which is depicted in **Fig. 7**. Infants with a high clinical risk score are at high risk for sepsis irrespective of their HRCi, and those with a high-risk HRCi (>2-fold increase in risk) are at increased risk for sepsis irrespective of their clinical risk score. For infants with a clinical risk score or HRCi in the low-risk zone or intermediate-risk zone, the risk of sepsis can be best predicted based on knowledge of both scores.[8]

Other Factors that Might Alter HRCi

Gestational and chronologic ages are associated with changes in HRC. Among very premature infants, as compared with more mature infants, variability, as indexed by the standard deviation and sample entropy, is lower and sample asymmetry and HRCi are higher. With increasing postmenstrual age, sample entropy and sample asymmetry increase and HRCi decreases.[7] The authors' observations of more than 300 infants at the University of Virginia and Wake Forest University NICUs suggest that surgery, initiation of mechanical ventilation, and treatment with pancuronium or fentanyl are associated with an acute increase in HRCi, whereas treatment with dexamethasone is associated with an acute decrease. Initiation of dobutamine or dopamine is also associated with an acute increase in HRCi, which might be explained by the underlying condition for which a vasopressor is prescribed.

SUMMARY AND FUTURE DIRECTIONS

Sepsis occurs frequently in hospitalized infants and increases mortality risk, hospital costs, and the risk of long-term developmental impairments. Each of these outcomes

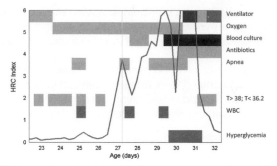

Fig. 8. Increased HRCi associated with sepsis. T, temperature; WBC, white blood cells.

might be improved by earlier identification and treatment of infants with sepsis. Continuous monitoring of the 3 time-based measures used to calculate HRC, such as standard deviation, sample asymmetry, and sample entropy, can be used to identify infants with sepsis before the development of clinical signs. An ongoing clinical trial might provide an answer to the question of whether continuous HRC monitoring can improve the outcome of hospitalized infants.

There is some evidence to suggest that the HRC accompanying sepsis, that is, transient heart rate decelerations and decreased variability, is associated with a systemic inflammatory response. Thus continuous HRC monitoring might provide a research tool for investigating the putative link between systemic inflammation and neurodevelopmental impairments and interventions to prevent inflammation-related brain damage in neonates.

APPENDIX 1: ILLUSTRATIVE CLINICAL CASE 1: INCREASED HRCI ASSOCIATED WITH SEPSIS

HRCi (red line) and clinical course (shaded boxes) of an infant born at 26-weeks' gestation. (Note: these HRCi data were recorded but not displayed to clinicians.) On day 27, the patient had apnea and leukocytosis. A blood culture that day showed no growth, but a repeat blood culture on day 29 yielded coagulase-negative *Staphylococcus*. On day 30, the patient required endotracheal intubation and mechanical ventilation and antibiotics were started. Note that over the 12 hours before the episode of apnea and the first blood culture on day 27, the HRCi increased from

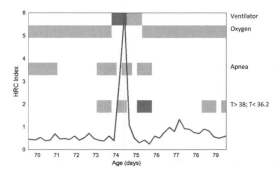

Fig. 9. Increased HRCi associated with surgical procedure. T, temperature.

a level of about 0.5, signifying a lower-than-average risk of sepsis, to a nearly 4-fold risk of sepsis. It increased in the next several days but decreased after initiation of antibiotics. The shaded boxes indicate symptoms, laboratory tests, and interventions (**Fig. 8**).

APPENDIX 2: ILLUSTRATIVE CLINICAL CASE 2: INCREASED HRCI ASSOCIATED WITH SURGICAL PROCEDURE

HRCi findings and clinical course of an infant born at 26 weeks' gestation. On day 74, the patient had laser retinal photocoagulation under general anesthesia. HRC monitoring resumed after the procedure. Blood culture was not sent, and no antibiotics were given. A large transient increase in HRCi is a typical finding after the surgical procedures (**Fig. 9**).

REFERENCES

1. Stoll BJ, Hansen N, Fanaroff AA, et al. Late-onset sepsis in very low birth weight neonates: the experience of the NICHD Neonatal Research Network. Pediatrics 2002;110(2 Pt 1):285–91.
2. Bassler D, Stoll BJ, Schmidt B, et al. Using a count of neonatal morbidities to predict poor outcome in extremely low birth weight infants: added role of neonatal infection. Pediatrics 2009;123(1):313–8.
3. Moorman JR, Lake DE, Griffin MP. Heart rate characteristics monitoring for neonatal sepsis. IEEE Trans Biomed Eng 2006;53(1):126–32.
4. Griffin MP, Lake DE, Bissonette EA, et al. Heart rate characteristics: novel physiomarkers to predict neonatal infection and death. Pediatrics 2005;116(5): 1070–4.
5. Griffin MP, Lake DE, Moorman JR. Heart rate characteristics and laboratory tests in neonatal sepsis. Pediatrics 2005;115(4):937–41.
6. Cao H, Lake DE, Griffin MP, et al. Increased nonstationarity of neonatal heart rate before the clinical diagnosis of sepsis. Ann Biomed Eng 2004;32(2):233–44.
7. Griffin MP, O'Shea TM, Bissonette EA, et al. Abnormal heart rate characteristics preceding neonatal sepsis and sepsis-like illness. Pediatr Res 2003;53(6): 920–6.
8. Griffin MP, Lake DE, O'Shea TM, et al. Heart rate characteristics and clinical signs in neonatal sepsis. Pediatr Res 2007;61(2):222–7.
9. Griffin MP, Moorman JR. Toward the early diagnosis of neonatal sepsis and sepsis-like illness using novel heart rate analysis. Pediatrics 2001;107(1):97–104.
10. Gang Y, Malik M. Heart rate variability in critical care medicine. Curr Opin Crit Care 2002;8(5):371–5.
11. Mangoni ME, Nargeot J. Genesis and regulation of the heart automaticity. Physiol Rev 2008;88(3):919–82.
12. Goehler LE, Gaykema RP, Hansen MK, et al. Vagal immune-to-brain communication: a visceral chemosensory pathway. Auton Neurosci 2000;85(1–3):49–59.
13. Fairchild KD, Saucerman JJ, Raynor LL, et al. Endotoxin depresses heart rate variability in mice: cytokine and steroid effects. Am J Physiol Regul Integr Comp Physiol 2009;297(4):R1019–27.
14. Borovikova LV, Ivanova S, Zhang M, et al. Vagus nerve stimulation attenuates the systemic inflammatory response to endotoxin. Nature 2000;405(6785):458–62.
15. Tracey KJ. Physiology and immunology of the cholinergic antiinflammatory pathway. J Clin Invest 2007;117(2):289–96.

16. Bernik TR, Friedman SG, Ochani M, et al. Pharmacological stimulation of the cholinergic antiinflammatory pathway. J Exp Med 2002;195(6):781–8.
17. Parrish WR, Rosas-Ballina M, Gallowitsch-Puerta M, et al. Modulation of TNF release by choline requires alpha7 subunit nicotinic acetylcholine receptor-mediated signaling. Mol Med 2008;14(9–10):567–74.
18. Su X, Lee JW, Matthay ZA, et al. Activation of the alpha7 nAChR reduces acid-induced acute lung injury in mice and rats. Am J Respir Cell Mol Biol 2007; 37(2):186–92.
19. Su X, Matthay MA, Malik AB. Requisite role of the cholinergic alpha7 nicotinic acetylcholine receptor pathway in suppressing gram-negative sepsis-induced acute lung inflammatory injury. J Immunol 2010;184(1):401–10.
20. Nizri E, Irony-Tur-Sinai M, Lory O, et al. Activation of the cholinergic anti-inflammatory system by nicotine attenuates neuroinflammation via suppression of Th1 and Th17 responses. J Immunol 2009;183(10):6681–8.
21. Saul JP, Berger RD, Albrecht P, et al. Transfer function analysis of the circulation: unique insights into cardiovascular regulation. Am J Physiol 1991;261(4 Pt 2): H1231–45.
22. Senat MV, Minoui S, Multon O, et al. Effect of dexamethasone and betamethasone on fetal heart rate variability in preterm labour: a randomised study. Br J Obstet Gynaecol 1998;105(7):749–55.
23. Morris JA Jr, Norris PR, Waitman LR, et al. Adrenal insufficiency, heart rate variability, and complex biologic systems: a study of 1,871 critically ill trauma patients. J Am Coll Surg 2007;204(5):885–92 [discussion: 892–3].
24. Aboab J, Polito A, Orlikowski D, et al. Hydrocortisone effects on cardiovascular variability in septic shock: a spectral analysis approach. Crit Care Med 2008; 36(5):1481–6.
25. Rajendra AU, Paul N, Kannathal C, et al. Heart rate variability: a review. Med Biol Eng Comput 2006;44(12):1031–51.
26. Heart rate variability: standards of measurement, physiological interpretation and clinical use. Task Force of the European Society of Cardiology and the North American Society of Pacing and Electrophysiology. Circulation 1996;93(5): 1043–65.
27. Chang KL, Monahan KJ, Griffin MP, et al. Comparison and clinical application of frequency domain methods in analysis of neonatal heart rate time series. Ann Biomed Eng 2001;29(9):764–74.
28. Griffin MP, Scollan DF, Moorman JR. The dynamic range of neonatal heart rate variability. J Cardiovasc Electrophysiol 1994;5(2):112–24.
29. Cao H, Lake DE, Ferguson JE 2nd, et al. Toward quantitative fetal heart rate monitoring. IEEE Trans Biomed Eng 2006;53(1):111–8.
30. Salafia CM, Ghidini A, Sherer DM, et al. Abnormalities of the fetal heart rate in preterm deliveries are associated with acute intra-amniotic infection. J Soc Gynecol Investig 1998;5(4):188–91.
31. Duff P, Sanders R, Gibbs RS. The course of labor in term patients with chorioamnionitis. Am J Obstet Gynecol 1983;147(4):391–5.
32. Goldstein B, Ellenby MS. Heart rate variability and critical illness: potential and problems. Crit Care Med 2000;28(12):3939–40.
33. Biswas AK, Scott WA, Sommerauer JF, et al. Heart rate variability after acute traumatic brain injury in children. Crit Care Med 2000;28(12):3907–12.
34. Hanna BD, Nelson MN, White-Traut RC, et al. Heart rate variability in preterm brain-injured and very-low-birth-weight infants. Biol Neonate 2000;77(3): 147–55.

35. Althaus JE, Petersen SM, Fox HE, et al. Can electronic fetal monitoring identify preterm neonates with cerebral white matter injury? Obstet Gynecol 2005; 105(3):458–65.
36. Goldstein B, Toweill D, Lai S, et al. Uncoupling of the autonomic and cardiovascular systems in acute brain injury. Am J Physiol 1998;275(4 Pt 2):R1287–92.
37. Thayer JF, Sternberg E. Beyond heart rate variability: vagal regulation of allostatic systems. Ann N Y Acad Sci 2006;1088:361–72.
38. Brown AD, Barton DA, Lambert GW. Cardiovascular abnormalities in patients with major depressive disorder: autonomic mechanisms and implications for treatment. CNS Drugs 2009;23(7):583–602.
39. Cohen H, Matar MA, Kaplan Z, et al. Power spectral analysis of heart rate variability in psychiatry. Psychother Psychosom 1999;68(2):59–66.
40. Alvarez SM, Katsamanis KM, Coyle SM, et al. Low-dose steroid alters in vivo endotoxin-induced systemic inflammation but does not influence autonomic dysfunction. J Endotoxin Res 2007;13(6):358–68.
41. Chen WL, Chen JH, Huang CC, et al. Heart rate variability measures as predictors of in-hospital mortality in ED patients with sepsis. Am J Emerg Med 2008; 26(4):395–401.
42. Ellenby MS, McNames J, Lai S, et al. Uncoupling and recoupling of autonomic regulation of the heart beat in pediatric septic shock. Shock 2001;16(4):274–7.
43. Dunser MW, Hasibeder WR. Sympathetic overstimulation during critical illness: adverse effects of adrenergic stress. J Intensive Care Med 2009;24(5):293–316.
44. Annane D, Trabold F, Sharshar T, et al. Inappropriate sympathetic activation at onset of septic shock: a spectral analysis approach. Am J Respir Crit Care Med 1999;160(2):458–65.
45. Boillot A, Massol J, Maupoil V, et al. Alterations of myocardial and vascular adrenergic receptor-mediated responses in Escherichia coli-induced septic shock in the rat. Crit Care Med 1996;24(8):1373–80.
46. Jones SB, Romano FD. Myocardial beta adrenergic receptor coupling to adenylate cyclase during developing septic shock. Circ Shock 1990;30(1):51–61.
47. Haensel A, Mills PJ, Nelesen RA, et al. The relationship between heart rate variability and inflammatory markers in cardiovascular diseases. Psychoneuroendocrinology 2008;33(10):1305–12.
48. Jan BU, Coyle SM, Macor MA, et al. Relationship of basal heart rate variability to in vivo cytokine responses following endotoxin. Shock 2009. [Epub ahead of print].
49. Tateishi Y, Oda S, Nakamura M, et al. Depressed heart rate variability is associated with high IL-6 blood level and decline in the blood pressure in septic patients. Shock 2007;28(5):549–53.
50. Papaioannou VE, Dragoumanis C, Theodorou V, et al. Relation of heart rate variability to serum levels of C-reactive protein, interleukin 6, and 10 in patients with sepsis and septic shock. J Crit Care 2009;24(4):625 e1–7.
51. Psychari SN, Sinos L, Latrou C, et al. Relations of inflammatory markers to lipid levels and autonomic tone in patients with moderate and severe chronic kidney disease and in patients under maintenance hemodialysis. Clin Nephrol 2005; 64(6):419–27.
52. Sloan RP, McCreath H, Tracey KJ, et al. RR interval variability is inversely related to inflammatory markers: the CARDIA study. Mol Med 2007;13(3–4):178–84.
53. Werdan K, Muller-Werdan U. Elucidating molecular mechanisms of septic cardiomyopathy—the cardiomyocyte model. Mol Cell Biochem 1996;163–4, 291–303.

54. Rudolph AJ, Vallbona C, Desmond MM. Cardiodynamic studies in the newborn. 3. Heart rate patterns in infants with idiopathic respiratory distress syndrome. Pediatrics 1965;36(4):551–9.
55. Cabal LA, Siassi B, Zanini B, et al. Factors affecting heart rate variability in preterm infants. Pediatrics 1980;65(1):50–6.
56. Richardson DK, Shah BL, Frantz ID 3rd, et al. Perinatal risk and severity of illness in newborns at 6 neonatal intensive care units. Am J Public Health 1999;89(4): 511–6.
57. Kovatchev BP, Farhy LS, Cao H, et al. Sample asymmetry analysis of heart rate characteristics with application to neonatal sepsis and systemic inflammatory response syndrome. Pediatr Res 2003;54(6):892–8.
58. Lake DE, Richman JS, Griffin MP, et al. Sample entropy analysis of neonatal heart rate variability. Am J Physiol Regul Integr Comp Physiol 2002;283(3):R789–97.
59. Griffin MP, O'Shea TM, Bissonette EA, et al. Abnormal heart rate characteristics are associated with neonatal mortality. Pediatr Res 2004;55(5):782–8.
60. Addison K, Griffin MP, Moorman JR, et al. Heart rate characteristics and neurodevelopmental outcome in very low birth weight infants. J Perinatol 2009; 29(11):750–6.

Biomarkers for Late-Onset Neonatal Sepsis: Cytokines and Beyond

Pak C. Ng, MD, FRCPCH*, Hugh S. Lam, MRCPCH

KEYWORDS
- Biomarkers • Infection • Infants • Late-onset

Early and accurate diagnosis of late-onset neonatal sepsis (LONS) is a major diagnostic challenge in neonatology.[1,2] LONS occurs most frequently in preterm and very low-birth-weight (VLBW) infants and in newborns with surgical conditions that require prolonged parenteral nutrition and hospitalization in the neonatal intensive care unit (NICU). A recent multicenter survey suggests that more than one-fifth (21%) of VLBW infants have at least 1 episode of late-onset culture-proven sepsis.[2] To date, clinical differentiation between LONS, including septicemia, meningitis, and systemic infection/inflammation (eg, necrotizing enterocolitis [NEC]), and noninfectious conditions (eg, acute exacerbation of bronchopulmonary dysplasia, apnea of prematurity, and gastrointestinal dysmotility) remains difficult, if not impossible, at an early stage of the illness.[1,3] A test or biomarker, which can accurately identify active infection/inflammation including septicemia and NEC in these vulnerable patients, would provide invaluable information for diagnosis and management. This review focuses on (1) the properties of an "ideal" diagnostic marker (or panel of biomarkers) of infection, (2) different categories of inflammatory mediators, such as acute phase proteins, chemokines, cytokines, and cell-surface antigens, that could potentially be used as clinical biomarkers, and (3) the use of molecular and biogenetic techniques for identification of pathogens in sterile body fluids. The authors also discuss recent scientific advances to search for novel biomarkers of infection in newborns.

THE IDEAL BIOMARKER OR TEST FOR LONS

The authors have previously proposed a set of clinical and laboratory criteria to assist neonatologists in identifying the ideal diagnostic marker of infection.[1] Although the

Financial disclosure: The authors do not have any financial disclosure.
Department of Pediatrics, Prince of Wales Hospital, The Chinese University of Hong Kong, Hong Kong
* Corresponding author. Department of Pediatrics, Level 6, Clinical Sciences Building, Prince of Wales Hospital, 30-32 Ngan Shing Street, Shatin, New Territories, Hong Kong.
E-mail address: pakcheungng@cuhk.edu.hk

Clin Perinatol 37 (2010) 599–610
doi:10.1016/j.clp.2010.05.005
0095-5108/10/$ – see front matter © 2010 Elsevier Inc. All rights reserved.

fundamental principles remain unchanged, with continuing advances in technology, neonatologists now expect more clinical information to be provided by biomarkers. **Box 1** summarizes current views on the characteristics of the ideal biomarker. The biomarker should not only serve as a guide on when to stop antimicrobial treatment in noninfected infants but also aid in the decision of whether to start antibiotic treatment at the onset of nonspecific clinical signs. With advances in molecular biogenetic techniques, the ideal biomarker or test is also expected to pinpoint precisely the identity or category of microorganism causing sepsis.[4] Information on the severity of infection and likelihood of progression to disseminated intravascular coagulation (DIC) would also provide invaluable insights to clinicians for targeting infants with sepsis who are most in need of urgent treatment and intensive care support.[5] Identification of the pathogen and antibiotic susceptibility profile at disease onset would also contribute enormously to acute management.

Box 1
The ideal biomarker or test for LONS

Clinical properties

1. Provide an algorithm for starting and/or stopping antimicrobial treatment. Such biomarkers should have

   - A well-defined cutoff value

   - A sensitivity and negative predictive value approaching 100% for "ruling out" LONS (but simultaneously having high specificity and positive predictive value >85%)

Note: A biomarker or test with very high specificity and positive predictive value can be used for ruling in sepsis

2. Detect infection early (ie, at clinical presentation)

3. Identify a specific pathogen or a category of pathogens (eg, viral, bacterial, and fungal organisms; gram-positive organisms vs gram-negative organisms; a specific species of pathogen)

4. Monitor disease progress and guide antimicrobial treatment (eg, bacterial antibiotic resistance gene detection)

5. Predict the disease severity at the onset of infection (eg, identify the type of virulent pathogen, predict DIC at the onset of disease presentation)

6. Predict prognosis (ie, mortality)

Laboratory properties

1. Stable compound that may allow an adequate time window for specimen collection within normal working hours (ie, sustained increase or decrease in biomarker level for at least 24 hours) or easy storage of the specimen without significant decomposition of the active compound until laboratory processing

2. Quantitative determination of biomarker concentration

3. Automatic and easy method of measurement

4. Quick turnaround time (ie, specimen collection, transport, laboratory processing time, and reporting of results to clinicians within 6 hours)

5. Small volume of specimen (ie, <0.5 mL blood)

6. Daily or on-demand availability of testing in clinical laboratories

7. Low-cost test that can be used as a routine measurement

Biochemically, a biomarker should be stable and remain significantly upregulated or downregulated in the body fluid compartment for at least 12 to 24 hours even after commencement of appropriate antimicrobial treatment. This would increase the chance of a true positive test result, given the variability of timing of testing relative to onset of disease and treatment. The ideal biomarker would be resistant to decomposition during transport and storage so that the result would accurately reflect the infant's clinical condition at the time of specimen sampling. Other properties listed in **Box 1** are also crucial for maximizing the utility of a biomarker as a routine diagnostic test in the NICU setting.

NONSPECIFIC BIOMARKERS OF LONS

To date, most of the biomarkers investigated are key proinflammatory or antiinflammatory mediators of the infection/inflammatory cascade. A major disadvantage of nonspecific biomarkers is their tendency to be influenced by inflammatory conditions that are not induced by sepsis, such as tissue injury and surgery. Furthermore, localized infections frequently escape detection. The discovery of new biomarkers is key because blood culture, the current gold standard for diagnosing septicemia, is suboptimal in newborn infants. False-negative results are common because of the small volume of blood sample and the intermittent presence and low density of circulating pathogens during the early stages of infection. Pretreatment with antibiotics further exacerbates this problem. Hematologic tests, such as the total white cell count, differential white cell count, immature to total neutrophil (I/T) ratio, white cell morphology, platelet count, and various hematologic scores, are in general not considered to be particularly useful for differentiating between sepsis/NEC and noninfectious conditions.[6–8] These hematologic tests have insufficient sensitivity and specificity to guide clinical management, in particular, antibiotic treatment.[1] Hematologic tests such as the I/T ratio are also suboptimal because of their complex methodology and requirement of skillful technicians to identify immature neutrophil forms on a peripheral blood smear.[1,6] Although the presence of neutropenia and thrombocytopenia are suggestive of severe systemic infection, other noninfectious conditions such as severe lung disease can cause thrombocytopenia because of platelet sequestration.[9] Because hematologic parameters have limited diagnostic utility, recent studies of biomarkers have concentrated on 3 major categories of mediators: (1) acute phase proteins, (2) chemokines and pro- and antiinflammatory cytokines, and (3) cell-surface antigens.

Acute Phase Proteins

Of the acute phase proteins, C-reactive protein (CRP), serum amyloid A (SAA), and procalcitonin (PCT) are the most extensively studied. CRP is widely used in many NICUs for diagnosis and monitoring of treatment in LONS and NEC.[10–12] It has been previously reported that CRP is a late biomarker with high specificity for neonatal sepsis.[10] The concentration of serum CRP is usually not elevated at the time of clinical presentation but is delayed by 6 to 8 hours after onset of symptoms.[10] Although CRP is generally considered a nonspecific biomarker, research has shown that it has high specificity for neonatal systemic infection because preterm infants have a narrow spectrum of disease compared with older patients. Noninfectious inflammatory conditions that can confound the diagnosis of sepsis in adult patients, such as rheumatoid arthritis, other connective tissue diseases, and inflammatory bowel disease, occur rarely in neonates. Therefore, significant increases in serum CRP concentrations are more likely to be associated with systemic sepsis or bowel inflammation/necrosis secondary to NEC. Serial measurements of CRP concentrations are particularly useful in ruling out sepsis, and persistently normal levels for 48 hours can assist in decision making for discontinuation of antibiotic treatment in infants with an equivocal presentation.[13] There are limitations to the application of measuring CRP levels because both false-positive and false-negative results have been reported. Importantly, the test is not sensitive in diagnosing localized infections such as pneumonia, urinary tract infection, and isolated low-grade fungal central nervous system infection.[14] It is also not a useful indicator after surgery or recent immunization because the circulating levels tend to be significantly elevated after these events.[1]

A study by Arnon and colleagues[15] comparing SAA with CRP and interleukin (IL)-6 suggested that SAA had higher sensitivity within the first 24 hours than the other 2 biomarkers for identification of LONS. In particular, the sensitivity of CRP was much worse during the early phase of infection, whereas IL-6 was suboptimal 24 hours after the onset.[10] The specificity of SAA was comparable to CRP throughout the clinical course. In addition, another study performed by the same investigators indicated that the mortality in infected preterm infants was inversely correlated with circulating SAA at 8 hours and at 24 hours.[16] These studies suggest that SAA may be a better biomarker than CRP and provide vital information on prognosis early in the course of infection.[16]

PCT has also been extensively studied in newborns and adults. The kinetics of PCT suggest that its serum concentration begins to increase 2 to 4 hours after exposure to bacterial products, peaks at 6 to 8 hours, and remains elevated for at least 24 hours. There is a physiologic increase in PCT levels during the first 48 hours of life, thought to be secondary to gastrointestinal bacterial colonization and subsequent translocation of endotoxin through the bowel wall.[17,18] However, the substantial increase in serum PCT concentration during bacterial infection can be easily differentiated from this minor physiologic increase during the immediate postnatal period.[18] Overall, the diagnostic utilities are similar to other acute phase reactants, although some studies have suggested that PCT may be superior with better sensitivity and specificity for identifying LONS.[18,19]

Other acute phase reactants and proteins, such as haptoglobin, lactoferrin, neopterin, inter-α-inhibitor proteins (IαIps),[20,21] lipopolysaccharide-binding protein (LBP),[22,23] and components of the complement pathways (eg, C5a, C5L2),[24,25] have been reported to be potentially useful diagnostic biomarkers. Particular interest has been focused on LBP and IαIps. LBP can theoretically fill in the diagnostic gap between the early (eg, IL-6) and the late biomarkers (eg, CRP) because of its chemical kinetics. A recent study has demonstrated that LBP was superior in sensitivity and negative predictive value compared with PCT, IL-6, and CRP for diagnosing neonatal infection.[23] Infected infants have also been shown to have significantly lower IαIp levels than noninfected infants.[20,21] Nonetheless, the latter studies on IαIp are relatively small and the clinical usefulness of those markers cannot be confirmed at this time. Based on current evidence and the availability of tests in clinical laboratories, most NICUs currently rely on serial measurements of CRP concentration for the identification of infants with LONS.

Chemokines and Cytokines

Chemokines and cytokines have been extensively studied in the past decade. Of this important category of mediators, the proinflammatory cytokine IL-6, the antiinflammatory cytokine IL-10, and chemokines IL-8, IP-10 (10-kDa interferon-γ-inducible protein), and RANTES (regulated upon activation, normal T cell expressed and secreted) have been found to be potentially useful for early diagnosis of LONS and for predicting the severity of infection at the onset of sepsis presentation.[5,10,26]

Proinflammatory mediators are early warning biomarkers because their circulating levels are rapidly and substantially increased after infection.[26,27] Because IL-6 induces the production of CRP in the liver, it is not surprising that its upregulation precedes that of CRP during sepsis.[10] The measurement of IL-6 in conjunction with IL-1 receptor antagonist (IL-1ra) may help predict LONS 2 days before clinical manifestations become evident.[28] IL-1ra has a longer half-life compared with other cytokines, potentially increasing its utility as a sepsis biomarker. IL-6 has a short half-life, and circulating levels decrease precipitously back to the baseline noninfectious state within 24 hours of appropriate treatment.[10] IL-8 (a chemokine) follows a similar time course. This characteristic greatly limits the role of IL-6 and IL-8 as clinically useful biomarkers across all phases of sepsis, although they may have utility in the early presentation before therapy. The quantitation of intracellular IL-8 by treating whole blood samples with detergent to lyse white blood cells may lengthen the window of opportunity for obtaining blood samples and further enhance the diagnostic utility.[29] Other chemokines and cytokines, such as tumor necrosis factor (TNF) α, monokine induced by interferon-γ, monocyte chemoattractant protein (MCP)-1, and growth-related oncogene α, are significantly upregulated during infection and NEC, whereas RANTES is downregulated, in some cases because of concomitant thrombocytopenia.[27] The utility of these diagnostic biomarkers is not as promising as those mentioned earlier.[27]

Another important group of inflammatory mediators is the antiinflammatory cytokines, such as IL-10 and transforming growth factor β, which are important in preventing an exaggerated proinflammatory response during sepsis.[30] An elevated antiinflammatory (IL-10) to proinflammatory (TNF-α) ratio in adult patients with infection has been associated with adverse outcomes.[31] Increased IL-10/TNF-α ratio has also been associated with severe LONS in VLBW infants.[32] In another study, an algorithm using sequential measurements of IL-10, IL-6, and RANTES at clinical presentation was shown to sensitively and reliably predict the development of DIC in severely infected infants.[5] This information is crucial for identifying seriously ill infants who are most in need of urgent treatment and intensive care support and may also assist in counseling of parents at a very early stage of illness. The magnitude and balance (or imbalance) of proinflammatory and antiinflammatory responses are a crucial reflection of the severity of sepsis and may play an important role in predicting morbidity and mortality.[5,31,32] Despite the favorable properties of chemokines and cytokines, assessment using these mediators has not been successfully integrated into routine clinical practice. High-cost, nonautomated, labor-intensive methodology and the lack of on-demand testing in clinical laboratories are major obstacles that have prevented the evolution of cytokines as routine diagnostic tests in the NICU setting.

Cell-surface Antigens

Advances in flow cytometric technology have paved the way to easy detection of cell-surface antigens on circulating inflammatory cells, including neutrophils, lymphocytes, monocytes, and natural killer (NK) cells. Specific cell-surface antigens are expressed in large quantities soon after the target cells are activated by microbial products and bacterial toxins.[3] Many cell-surface antigens have been investigated in relation to neonatal sepsis,[33] and the most promising ones are neutrophil CD64[34–36] and neutrophil/monocyte CD11b.[37–39]

CD64 and CD11b are antigens that are expressed at very low densities on nonactivated white blood cell surfaces. During bacterial and fungal infection or NEC, these antigens are substantially upregulated and their concentrations on the cell surface can be accurately and quantitatively measured by flow cytometry. The authors' findings suggest that neutrophil CD64 is a sensitive biomarker for diagnosis of early-onset sepsis and LONS,[34–36] and its upregulation significantly precedes that of CRP. Recently, neutrophil CD64 has also been demonstrated to be a good indicator of intra-abdominal sepsis, including NEC, bowel perforation, and peritonitis. As expected, this test is unable to differentiate between systemic infection and intra-abdominal sepsis/inflammation (Lam HS and colleagues, unpublished data, 2010). Neutrophil CD11b has also been suggested to be a sensitive biomarker for early-onset neonatal infection,[37,38] and a subsequent study on daily surveillance showed that neutrophil/monocyte CD11b could reveal evidence of infection up to 3 days before clinical manifestations.[39] Such findings have not been repeated and would require validation by larger studies. Unlike with CD64, the results with CD11b are more variable, and the findings have not been consistent between centers.[34] Expression of CD11b is also influenced by noninfectious conditions such as respiratory distress syndrome.[40] The authors have compared neutrophil CD64 and neutrophil CD11b within the same study and found that CD64 had significantly better utility than CD11b in diagnosing LONS and NEC.[34] Other cell-surface antigens, including NK cell CD69,[41] lymphocyte CD25 and CD45RO,[34] and an elaborate panel of leukocyte surface antigens including CD19, CD33, and CD66b, have also been investigated,[33] but none showed better diagnostic utility than CD64 and CD11b. Advantages of flow cytometry include small blood volume (50 μL whole blood), rapid turnaround time (<4 hours), wide window of opportunity for blood sampling, and ability to perform the test on an ad hoc basis. The disadvantage is that flow cytometry requires skilled technicians to carry out multistep measurements semiautomatically, and flow cytometry is not considered a routine diagnostic evaluation in most NICUs.

Quantitative Polymerase Chain Reaction

The quantitative polymerase chain reaction (qPCR) is a rapid test that can detect bacterial DNA in sterile body fluids, including blood and pleural, peritoneal, and cerebrospinal fluid, and is most desirable when conventional microbiologic methods fail to detect organisms. Molecular techniques such as fluorescence in situ hybridization can substantially reduce the time required to identify organisms isolated in culture.[42] This reduction can be as much as 18 hours for bacterial isolates and 42 hours for yeasts.[42] Directly detecting pathogen DNA is attractive, especially when the target is a fastidious or slow-growing organism. Molecular techniques that focus on identification of a single species of bacteria are not particularly useful in an intensive care setting. An ideal test would encompass a wide variety of pathogens commonly encountered in NICUs. The use of the probe-based gram-specific qPCR for rapid detection and differentiation of gram-negative and gram-positive bloodstream infections has been attempted in recent studies.[4,43] This test has very high specificity and positive predictive value, especially for identification of gram-negative organisms.[4,43] Although the test is not sensitive enough for ruling out sepsis, it is particularly useful for ruling in sepsis because of its high specificity. Thus, a positive test result would strongly indicate the need for a full course of antimicrobial treatment despite negative culture of pathogens.[4] The identification of gram-specific sepsis would serve as a useful guide for prescribing appropriate and effective antibiotics and predicting the virulence of the causative pathogens and severity of infection.[4,43] The major limitations identified in these studies are (1) uncommon organisms not included in the genetic sequence of the primer/probes would escape detection and (2) gram-positive organisms and fungi with elaborate cell wall structures are resilient to digestion and destruction, posing a major problem for DNA extraction.[4] Use of molecular diagnostics for detecting bloodstream infections in neonates has shown some promise and some technical challenges.[44]

Identification of Resistance Genes by Molecular Techniques

The time required for conventional methods to isolate pathogens results in a significant delay of at least several days before vital information on antibiotic sensitivity becomes available. Recently, investigators using microarray-based techniques have demonstrated the possibility of detecting bacterial antibiotic resistance genes within a few hours.[45,46] Studies aiming to identify genes encoding resistance to first-line antibiotics are critically important when choosing empiric therapy in infants with suspected sepsis.

Genomics

Concentrations of cytokines and chemokines within the bloodstream often do not fully reflect the infective or inflammatory process that is ongoing within the patient.[1] Recently, investigators have focused on the possibility of identifying genes that are upregulated in infection. One study measuring whole blood IL-8 and MCP-1 mRNA concentrations suggested that levels of both mRNAs were elevated in infants with perinatal asphyxia, whereas only IL-8 mRNA level was elevated in infants with perinatal infection.[47] The detection of tissue-specific mRNA could potentially be used as a basis for developing disease-specific biomarkers in neonates.

Proteomics

Mass spectrometry–based proteomic profiling technologies, such as surface-enhanced laser desorption/ionization, have been used to identify host response proteins as signatures for diagnosis of a wide variety of pathologic conditions and diseases, such as severe acute respiratory syndrome, intra-amniotic inflammation, and neonatal sepsis.[48] To date, all clinical studies involving acute phase proteins, chemokines, cytokines, and cell-surface antigens selected key mediators or antigens in the infection/inflammatory cascade, using the traditional "candidate" approach, and tested their diagnostic utility for LONS. This conventional approach greatly confines and restricts the search for biomarkers to known mediators or proteins of the cascade. In contrast, the proteomics technology with its "hypothesis-free" approach can potentially discover novel host response biomarkers for diagnosis of LONS and NEC in preterm infants. The authors recently completed a proteomics project and discovered one known protein and one novel lipoprotein for early and accurate identification of infants with sepsis and NEC.[49] A new proteomics sepsis score derived from these two biomarkers would guide frontline neonatologists whether to 'start' antibiotic treatment at the time of clinical presentation and to 'stop' therapy within 24 hours of commencement. This score ensures patient safety with 100% negative predictive value. It would preclude a significant proportion (>60%) of true non-sepsis cases from receiving antibiotics unnecessarily or for very early withdrawal of treatment. The proteomics technology may further assist in identifying novel biochemical pathways associated with infection. It is a powerful tool for biomarker discovery, and we have demonstrated that the technology can be competently applied to very premature infants. A limitation of proteomics is that proteins with low plasma concentrations, such as chemokines and cytokines, may not be easily detected by this method. In addition, a stringent protocol with elaborate study design is required to ensure that the proteins identified are genuinely representative and specific for the condition investigated.

SUMMARY AND FUTURE CONSIDERATIONS

To date, no single "ideal" diagnostic biomarker of LONS has been identified. **Table 1** summarizes the pros and cons of different categories of inflammatory mediators and

Table 1
Advantages and disadvantages of diagnostic biomarkers and tests for LONS

Diagnostic Tests	Diagnostic Utilities	Identification of Specific Pathogens or Conditions	Prediction of Severity and/or Prognosis	Monitoring Progress	Ruling Out vs Ruling in Sepsis	Timing of Specimen Collection	Turnaround Time (h)[b]
Hematologic Tests							
Simple (eg, WCC, differential WCC, I/T ratio, platelets)	Poor	Nonspecific	Fair (neutropenia and DIC in severe sepsis)	Poor	Neither	Any time	4–6
Complex (eg, hematologic scores)	Fair	Nonspecific	?[a]	Poor	Neither	Any time	8–17
Acute Phase Proteins (eg, CRP, SAA)	Good	Nonspecific	Good (higher levels in severe sepsis)	Good	Ruling out	Late	4–6
Chemokines/ Cytokines (eg, IP-10, IL-6, IL-8, IL-10, RANTES)	Very good	Nonspecific	Good (higher levels in severe sepsis)	?[a]	Ruling out	Early	4–6[c]
Leukocyte Surface Antigens (eg, CD64, CD11b)	Very good	Nonspecific	Good (higher levels in severe sepsis)	Fair	Ruling out	Early and late	4[c]
qPCR (eg, gram-specific gene probe)	Very good (gram-negative organisms), fair (gram-positive organisms)	Specific (especially gram-negative organisms)	?[a] (uncertain association with circulating gene copies)	Poor	Ruling in	Early	8–17[c]

Blood Volume (mL)	Test Availability	Measurement			Comments	Routine/ Experimental
		Quantitative (Q)/ Semiquantitative (S-Q)	Automatic Measurement	Low Cost		
0.5–1.0	On demand	Q	Y	Y	DIC	Routine
0.5–1.0	On demand	S-Q	N	?[a]	—	Hematologic score rarely performed
0.5–1.0	On demand	Q	Y	Y	Late biomarker Serial CRP for ruling out sepsis and early stoppage of antibiotics Monitor disease progress	Routine in many NICUs
0.1–0.2 per mediator	Batches	Q	N	N	Early biomarker Predict DIC at the onset Prognostication Multiplex technology for many analytes on small blood volume	Experimental
0.05	On demand	Q or S-Q	N	N	Early biomarker	Selected cases/ experimental
1.0	On demand	Q or S-Q[d]	N	N	Early diagnosis Especially useful in culture-negative cases	Selected cases (especially culture-negative cases)/ experimental

Abbreviations: IP, interferon-γ-inducible protein; N, no; WCC, white cell count; Y, yes.
[a] Uncertain association.
[b] Time from specimen collection to announcement of results.
[c] Tests not routinely available in most clinical laboratories.
[d] Gene copies can be measured.

tests that have been clinically evaluated. The ideal biomarker panel would provide information to facilitate early diagnosis and predict the severity of infection and outcomes at the onset of clinical signs and symptoms. For example, at first suspicion of sepsis, the proteomics sepsis score and early biomarkers, including neutrophil CD64, IL-6, and IL-10, could be used to decide whether to start antimicrobial treatment and also to give forewarning of the severity of sepsis and likelihood of development of DIC.[5,10,32,34,49] At 24 hours, a repeat proteomics sepsis score and neutrophil CD64 could facilitate the decision to discontinue antibiotics in nonsepsis cases.[34,49] Thereafter, serial CRP level measurements may be useful in monitoring the progress or development of late complications.[1,10,11] Molecular diagnostics could be considered for highly suspected cases of sepsis or NEC with negative blood culture[4] or for testing of other sterile body fluids to provide microbiologic information not obtainable by other nonspecific tests.

The clinical research team is primarily responsible for identifying favorable biomarkers and confirming the clinical and laboratory properties of these biomarkers in a typical hospital or NICU setting. One of the main reasons why most favorable biomarkers have not become routine clinical tests is because no automated method of measurement has been developed by the industrial sector. Academic-industry partnership is essential for successful development of new and clinically useful diagnostic biomarkers. Because new molecular and biogenetic technologies are rapidly advancing, nonspecific biomarkers would likely be replaced by more specific tests, which could pinpoint the precise condition (ie, differentiating between septicemia and NEC or focal infections such as pneumonia) and provide vital information on the pathogen and its antibiotic resistance profile within hours of clinical presentation.

REFERENCES

1. Ng PC. Diagnostic markers of infection in neonates. Arch Dis Child Fetal Neonatal Ed 2004;89(3):229–35.
2. Stoll BJ, Hansen N, Fanaroff AA, et al. Late-onset sepsis in very low birth weight neonates: the experience of the NICHD Neonatal Research Network. Pediatrics 2002;110(2):285–91.
3. Lam HS, Ng PC. Biochemical markers of neonatal sepsis. Pathology 2008;40(2):141–8.
4. Chan KY, Lam HS, Cheung HM, et al. Rapid identification and differential of Gram-negative and Gram-positive bacterial bloodstream infections by quantitative polymerase chain reaction in preterm infants. Crit Care Med 2009;37(8):2441–7.
5. Ng PC, Li K, Leung TF, et al. Early prediction of sepsis-induced disseminated intravascular coagulation with interleukin-10, interleukin-6, and RANTES in preterm infants. Clin Chem 2006;52(6):1181–9.
6. Rodwell RL, Leslie AL, Tudehope DI. Early diagnosis of neonatal sepsis using a hematologic scoring system. J Pediatr 1988;112(5):761–7.
7. Howard MR, Smith RA. Early diagnosis of septicaemia in preterm infants from examination of peripheral blood films. Clin Lab Haematol 1999;21(5):365–8.
8. Da Silva O, Ohlsson A, Kenyon C. Accuracy of leukocyte indices and C-reactive protein for diagnosis of neonatal sepsis: a critical review. Pediatr Infect Dis J 1995;14(5):362–6.
9. Yang J, Yang M, Xu F, et al. Effects of oxygen-induced lung damage on megakaryocytopoiesis and platelet homeostasis in a rat model. Pediatr Res 2003;54(3):344–52.

10. Ng PC, Cheng SH, Chui KM, et al. Diagnosis of late onset neonatal sepsis with cytokines, adhesion molecule, and C-reactive protein in preterm very low birth weight infants. Arch Dis Child Fetal Neonatal Ed 1997;77(3):221–7.
11. Pourcyrous M, Korones SB, Yang W, et al. C-reactive protein in the diagnosis, management and prognosis of neonatal necrotizing enterocolitis. Pediatrics 2005;116(5):1064–9.
12. Philip AG, Mills PC. Use of C-reactive protein in minimizing antibiotic exposure: experience with infants initially admitted to a well-baby nursery. Pediatrics 2000;106(1):E4.
13. Polin RA. The 'ins and outs' of neonatal sepsis. J Pediatr 2003;143(1):3–4.
14. Ng PC, Lee CH, Fok TF, et al. Central nervous system candidiasis in preterm infants: limited value of biochemical markers for diagnosis. J Paediatr Child Health 2000;36(5):509–10.
15. Arnon S, Litmanovitz I, Regev R, et al. Serum amyloid A protein is a useful inflammatory marker during late-onset sepsis in preterm infants. Biol Neonate 2005; 87(2):105–10.
16. Arnon S, Litmanovitz I, Regev R, et al. The prognostic virtue of inflammatory markers during late-onset sepsis in preterm infants. J Perinat Med 2004;32(2): 176–80.
17. Dandona P, Nix D, Wilson MF, et al. Procalcitonin increase after endotoxin injection in normal subjects. J Clin Endocrinol Metab 1994;79(6):1605–8.
18. Chiesa C, Panero A, Rossi N, et al. Reliability of procalcitonin concentrations for the diagnosis of sepsis in critically ill neonates. Clin Infect Dis 1998;26(3):664–72.
19. Guibourdenche J, Bedu A, Petzold L, et al. Biochemical markers of neonatal sepsis: value of procalcitonin in the emergency setting. Ann Clin Biochem 2002;39(2):130–5.
20. Baek YW, Brokat S, Padbury JF, et al. Inter-alpha inhibitor proteins in infants and decreased levels in neonatal sepsis. J Pediatr 2003;143(1):11–5.
21. Lim YP, Bendelja K, Opal SM, et al. Correlation between mortality and the levels of inter-alpha inhibitors in the plasma of patients with severe sepsis. J Infect Dis 2003;188(6):919–26.
22. Behrendt D, Dembinski J, Heep A, et al. Lipopolysaccharide binding protein in preterm infants. Arch Dis Child Fetal Neonatal Ed 2004;89(6):551–4.
23. Pavcnik-Arnol M, Hojker S, Derganc M. Lipopolysaccharide-binding protein in critically ill neonates and children with suspected infection: comparison with procalcitonin, interleukin-6, and C-reactive protein. Intensive Care Med 2004;30(7):1454–60.
24. Ward PA. The dark side of C5a in sepsis. Nat Rev Immunol 2004;4(2):133–42.
25. Huber-Lang M, Sarma JV, Rittirsch D, et al. Changes in the novel orphan, C5a receptor (C5L2), during experimental sepsis and sepsis in humans. J Immunol 2005;174(2):1104–10.
26. Franz AR, Bauer K, Schalk A, et al. Measurement of interleukin 8 in combination with C-reactive protein reduced unnecessary antibiotic therapy in newborn infants: a multicenter, randomized, controlled trial. Pediatrics 2004;114(1):1–8.
27. Ng PC, Li K, Chui KM, et al. IP-10 is an early diagnostic marker for identification of late-onset bacterial infection in preterm infants. Pediatr Res 2007;61(1):93–8.
28. Küster H, Weiss M, Willeitner AE, et al. Interleukin-1 receptor antagonist and interleukin-6 for early diagnosis of neonatal sepsis 2 days before clinical manifestation. Lancet 1998;352(9136):1271–7.
29. Orlikowsky TW, Neunhoeffer F, Goelz R, et al. Evaluation of IL-8 concentrations in plasma and lysed EDTA-blood in healthy neonates and those with suspected early onset bacterial infection. Pediatr Res 2004;56(5):804–9.

30. Schultz C, Strunk T, Temming P, et al. Reduced IL-10 production and -receptor expression in neonatal T lymphocytes. Acta Paediatr 2007;96(8):1122–5.
31. van Dissel JT, van Langevelde P, Westendorp RG, et al. Anti-inflammatory cytokine profile and mortality in febrile patients. Lancet 1998;351(9107):950–3.
32. Ng PC, Li K, Wong RP, et al. Proinflammatory and anti-inflammatory cytokine responses in preterm infants with systemic infections. Arch Dis Child Fetal Neonatal Ed 2003;88(3):209–13.
33. Weinschenk NP, Farina A, Bianchi DW. Premature infants respond to early-onset and late-onset sepsis with leukocyte activation. J Pediatr 2000;137(3):345–50.
34. Ng PC, Li K, Wong RP, et al. Neutrophil CD64 expression: a sensitive diagnostic marker for late-onset nosocomial infection in very low birth weight infants. Pediatr Res 2002;51(3):296–303.
35. Ng PC, Li G, Chui KM, et al. Neutrophil CD64 is a sensitive diagnostic marker for early-onset neonatal infection. Pediatr Res 2004;56(5):796–803.
36. Bhandari V, Wang C, Rinder C, et al. Hematologic profile of sepsis in neonates: neutrophil CD64 as a diagnostic marker. Pediatrics 2008;121(1):129–34.
37. Weirich E, Rabin RL, Maldonado Y, et al. Neutrophil CD11b expression as a diagnostic marker for early-onset neonatal infection. J Pediatr 1998;132(3):445–51.
38. Nupponen I, Andersson S, Jarvenpaa AL, et al. Neutrophil CD11b expression and circulating interleukin-8 as diagnostic markers for early-onset neonatal sepsis. Pediatrics 2001;108(1):E12.
39. Turunen R, Andersson S, Nupponen I, et al. Increased CD11b-density on circulating phagocytes as an early sign of late-onset sepsis in extremely low-birth-weight infants. Pediatr Res 2005;57(2):270–5.
40. Nupponen I, Pesonen E, Andersson S, et al. Neutrophil activation in preterm infants who have respiratory distress syndrome. Pediatrics 2002;110(1):36–41.
41. Hodge G, Hodge S, Haslam R, et al. Rapid simultaneous measurement of multiple cytokines using 100 microl sample volumes—association with neonatal sepsis. Clin Exp Immunol 2004;137(2):402–7.
42. Wu YD, Chen LH, Wu XJ, et al. Gram stain-specific-probe-base real-time PCR for diagnosis and discrimination of bacterial neonatal sepsis. J Clin Microbiol 2008; 46(8):2613–9.
43. Peters RP, Savelkoul PH, Simoons-Smit AM, et al. Faster identification of pathogens in positive blood cultures by fluorescence in situ hybridization in routine practice. J Clin Microbiol 2006;44(1):119–23.
44. Jordan J. Molecular Diagnosis of Neonatal Sepsis. Clin Perinatol 2010;37(2): 411–9.
45. Perreten V, Vorlet-Fawer L, Slickers P, et al. Microarray-based detection of 90 antibiotic resistance genes of grampositive bacteria. J Clin Microbiol 2005;43(5): 2291–302.
46. Call DR, Bakko MK, Krug MJ, et al. Identifying antimicrobial resistance genes with DNA microarrays. Antimicrobial Agents Chemother 2003;47(10):3290–5.
47. Petrakou E, Mouchtouri A, Levi E, et al. Interleukin-8 and monocyte chemotactic protein-1 mRNA expression in perinatally infected and asphyxiated preterm neonates. Neonatology 2007;91(2):107–13.
48. Buhimschi I, Buhimschi C. The Role of Proteomics in the Diagnosis of Chorioamnionitis and Early-Onset Neonatal Sepsis. Clin Perinatol 2010;37(2):355–74.
49. Ng PC, Ang IL, Chiu RW, et al. Host-response biomarkers for diagnosis of late-onset septicemia and necrotizing enterocolitis in preterm infants. J Clin Invest 2010;120(8):2989–3000.

Strategies to Prevent Invasive Candidal Infection in Extremely Preterm Infants

David A. Kaufman, MD[a],*, Paolo Manzoni, MD[b]

KEYWORDS

- Preterm infants • Invasive candidal infection
- Antifungal prophylaxis • Fluconazole

IS IT POSSIBLE TO ELIMINATE INVASIVE CANDIDAL INFECTIONS FROM THE NEONATAL INTENSIVE CARE UNIT?

Case 1

An infant born at 25 weeks' gestation via vaginal delivery because of preterm labor is intubated and started on a feeding advance with breast milk. On day 23, he develops an ileus, new-onset thrombocytopenia, and hypotension and undergoes a sepsis evaluation. Cultures are sent and nafcillin and gentamicin begun. After 2 days of antibiotics, there is no growth from his cultures, yet he remains sick. Cultures are resent and *Candida albicans* is isolated from the blood. Treatment with amphotericin is administered for 4 weeks. He is discharged on day 110 and neurodevelopmental examination at 20 months demonstrates a Bayley Mental Developmental Index (MDI) of 68 (>2 standard deviations below the mean).

Case 2

An infant is born via spontaneous vaginal delivery at 24 weeks' gestation after premature rupture of membranes. She is intubated in the delivery room and umbilical catheters placed in the neonatal intensive care unit (NICU). Twice-weekly fluconazole prophylaxis is started on day 1. On day 4, a peripherally inserted central catheter (PICC) is placed and umbilical lines removed. Full enteral feeds are reached on day 24, the PICC is removed, and fluconazole prophylaxis is discontinued. She survives to discharge on day 90, with a normal Bayley MDI at 20 months.

[a] Division of Neonatology, Department of Pediatrics, University of Virginia School of Medicine, Box 800386 Charlottesville, VA 22903, USA
[b] Neonatology and NICU, Sant'Anna Hospital, C. Spezia, 60 - 10126 Torino, Italy
* Corresponding author.
E-mail address: dak4r@virginia.edu

Clin Perinatol 37 (2010) 611–628
doi:10.1016/j.clp.2010.06.003
0095-5108/10/$ – see front matter © 2010 Elsevier Inc. All rights reserved.

These scenarios illustrate the divergent courses of extremely preterm infants born in different NICUs. Currently, fluconazole prophylaxis is only offered in some NICUs, despite mounting evidence of its safety and efficacy. The pros and cons of antifungal prophylaxis are discussed in this article and a rational basis provided for neonatologists to make decisions about how to prevent these high-morbidity and -mortality infections.

INCIDENCE AND COMPLICATIONS OF INVASIVE CANDIDAL INFECTION

A significant issue in reviewing the literature on incidence, morbidity, and mortality of invasive candidal infection (ICI) in the NICU is the variability in reporting. *Candida* has a propensity for tissue invasion. Therefore, when signs of systemic infection exist, positive candidal cultures from normally sterile body fluids, including urine, cerebrospinal fluid (CSF), and peritoneal fluid, should be considered as an ICI. Also, each gestational age category should be considered in reporting incidence of ICI, because these infections are much more common among extremely preterm neonates. Another important consideration in reviewing the literature on *Candida* is whether treatment of infants with ICI was standardized and optimized, including removal of central vascular catheters. Regarding treatment, the specifics of agent, dose, route, and duration of treatment should also be taken into account. Whether or not antifungal agents were administered for prophylaxis must be considered. A final source of variability is that mortality is reported in various ways, including *Candida*-related, *Candida*-attributable (comparing infected to noninfected patients), and all-cause mortality.

The highest incidence of ICI occurs in the most extremely preterm infants (<1000 g birth weight and/or ≤27 weeks' gestation). Johnsson and colleagues[1] reported a rate of candidal bloodstream infection of 20% in infants aged 24 weeks and younger and 7% overall in infants with birth weight less than 1000 g. Fungal infections may be limited to the bloodstream, urine, or CSF or may disseminate to involve one or many organ systems. Fungal abscesses may be found in the heart, bones, kidneys, bladder, eye, or brain. There is a marked difference in mortality between infants weighing less than 1000 g and more mature infants with ICI. In infants weighing less than 1000 g with ICI, a recent analysis reported an all-cause mortality rate of 26% compared with 13% in infants without candidiasis. For infants greater than 1000 g with ICI, mortality was 2% compared with 0.4%.[2]

ICI may lead to significant neurodevelopmental impairment, even in absence of documented fungal meningitis. Some studies report an incidence of neurodevelopmental impairment of 57% in infected extremely low–birth-weight (ELBW) infants (<1000 g at birth) versus 29% in noninfected neonates.[2–6] Many factors contribute to neurodevelopmental impairment in ELBW infants, including shock, intraventricular hemorrhage, chronic lung disease, hypoxia, hyperoxia, apnea, postnatal steroids, necrotizing enterocolitis (NEC), focal bowel perforation, and bacterial and fungal infections. Sepsis, including ICI, involves a systemic inflammatory response, which may adversely affect the brain. Neonates with sepsis may also develop complications that increase risk of neurodevelopmental impairment, including hypotension and hypoxia, and of the need for more prolonged mechanical ventilation. Preventing neurodevelopmental impairment in high-risk ELBW infants involves a "bundle" strategy targeting all contributing factors, including antifungal prevention.

ANTIFUNGAL PROPHYLAXIS: EFFICACY AND SAFETY

The preterm infant is highly susceptible to infection from being immunocompromised and requiring invasive therapies. The developing immune system improves in function over time in the NICU as need for intensive care interventions (central venous and arterial catheters, parenteral nutrition, intubation, and antibiotics) decreases, making the highest risk period for infection the first 4 to 8 weeks of life. ICIs occur in immunocompromised patients, including neutropenic adults, most of whom are colonized with *Candida* at multiple sites. Prophylactic antifungal therapy has been shown to reduce ICI in these patients. In contrast to adults, most infants are not colonized or have low colony counts of yeast at birth, making them ideal candidates for antifungal prophylaxis. Prophylaxis is most effective at preventing or eradicating candidal colonization of the skin, gastrointestinal and respiratory tracts, and central venous catheter when started in the first day or two after birth.[7–10]

Fluconazole Prophylaxis in Extremely Preterm Neonates: Evidence from Clinical Trials

Fourteen studies of fluconazole prophylaxis in more than 4000 neonates have consistently demonstrated efficacy and safety, with an overall reduction in ICI of 83% and near elimination of *Candida*-related mortality (**Table 1**).[7,8,11–23,28] The overall incidence of ICI in the placebo or control (untreated) groups is 9% compared with 1.6% in the fluconazole prophylaxis groups ($P<.0001$). Subanalysis demonstrates that efficacy is highest (approximately 90%) in the smallest (<750 g or <1000 g) and youngest infants ($\leq$27 weeks). The safety of fluconazole prophylaxis and emergence of resistance have been detailed in recent reviews.[29] No significant adverse effects have been documented and no significant resistance has emerged with the use of prophylaxis.[7,8,11–23,28,30,31]

Three key randomized trials provide evidence of efficacy and safety of fluconazole prophylaxis.[7,8,11] The first study was a prospective, randomized, double-blind single-center trial involving 100 high-risk preterm infants with birth weight less than 1000 g who required central venous access or endotracheal intubation.[7] Infants were randomly assigned during the first 5 days of life to receive 3 mg/kg fluconazole intravenously (IV) or placebo for up to 6 weeks. None of the infants in the treatment group developed ICI compared with 20% of infants in the placebo group ($P = .008$). A subanalysis of infants of less than 24 weeks' gestational age (9% of the cohort) revealed that fluconazole treatment was efficacious even in the most immature of infants ($P = .04$).

In a subsequent randomized trial of fluconazole prophylaxis by the same group of investigators, the dosing schedule was studied, and 3 mg/kg administered twice weekly was as effective in preventing ICIs as the more frequent dosing schedule used in the previous study.[11] The twice-weekly dosing regimen reduced pharmacy and nursing time, drug costs and exposure and, possibly, the risk of development of azole resistance among fungi.

A multi-center, randomized, placebo-controlled trial investigating 2 different fluconazole doses (3 and 6 mg/kg) compared with placebo in infants with birth weight less than 1500 g (n = 322) confirmed the efficacy of fluconazole prophylaxis in preventing ICI.[8] The incidence of ICIs was decreased by 75% in both fluconazole dosing groups when compared with the placebo group (odds ratio [OR] 0.25; 95% confidence interval [CI], 0.10–0.59; $P = .001$). In a secondary analysis, prophylaxis was efficacious for infants of less than 27 weeks' gestational age ($P = .007$) and birth weight less than 1000 g ($P = .02$). Dosing with either 3 or 6 mg/kg had similar efficacy in decreasing colonization and ICIs. There were no adverse effects, and prophylaxis did not select drug-resistant strains during the study period. Additionally, there was no difference in the incidence of cholestasis or abnormal liver enzymes among the 3 groups.

Table 1
Invasive *Candida* infection prophylaxis studies in preterm infants

Fluconazole Prophylaxis: Randomized Controlled Studies

Study	n	ICI Incidence: Fluconazole	ICI Incidence: Placebo	P Value	Comments
Kaufman et al[7]	100	0 of 50 (0%)[a]	10 of 50 (20%)[a] / 4 *Candida*-related deaths	.008	<1000 g / Single center, placebo-control / 9% of infants in this study were <24 weeks old and highly effective (P = .04) in this group
Manzoni et al[8]	322	7 of 216 (3.2%)[a] / No *Candida*-related deaths	14 of 106 (13.2%)[a] / 2 *Candida*-related deaths	<.0001	<1500 g / Multicenter, placebo-control, 3-arm study
Kaufman et al[11]	81	2 of 41 (5%)[a] / More frequent dosing / vs / 1 of 40 (2.5%)[a] / Less frequent dosing / No *Candida*-related deaths	Dose comparison study. No placebo group	.68	<1000 g / Single center / Comparison of 2 dosing schedules. Less frequent dosing (3 mg/kg twice a week) is equally effective
Kicklighter et al[12]	103	1 of 53(1.9%)[a] / 1 *Candida*-related death	0 of 50 (0%)[a]	.52	<1500 g / Single center / Colonization study (1° endpoint)

Fluconazole Prophylaxis: Retrospective Studies with Historic Controls

Study	n	ICI Incidence: Fluconazole	ICI Incidence: Historic controls	P Value	Comments
Aghai et al[13]	277	0 of 140 (0%)[a]	9 of 137 (6.6%)[a] / 6 *Candida*-related deaths	.006	<1000 g (FP)
Manzoni et al[14]	465	4 of 225 (1.8%)[a] / No *Candida*-related deaths	22 of 240 (9.2%)[a] / 4 *Candida*-related deaths	.001	<1500 g
Bertini et al[15]	255	0 of 136 (0%)[a]	9 of 119 (7.6%)[a] / 3 *Candida*-related deaths	.003	<1500 g and CVC
Uko et al[16]	384	2 of 178 (1.1%)[a,b] / No *Candida*-related death	13 of 206 (6.3%)[a] / 2 *Candida*-related deaths	.007	<1500 g or <32 wks / Only during antibiotic administration of >3 d

Study	N			P value	Notes
Healy et al[17,18]	654	8 of 448 (1.8%)c No Candida-related deaths	15 of 206 (7%)c 4 Candida-related deaths	.003 .01	<1000 g FP significantly eliminated Candida-related mortality in entire NICU NEC and total parenteral nutrition days but not fluconazole prophylaxis were significantly associated with the development of cholestasis
Weitkamp et al[19]	86	0 of 42 (0)%a	9 of 44 (20%)a 1 Candida-related death	.004	<750 g or <26 wk and CVC Less empiric antifungal use after FP instituted
Aziz et al[20]	262	3 of 163 (1.8%)a 1 Candida-related death	7 of 99 (7.2%)a 1 Candida-related death	.045	<1000 g Cholestasis at discharge: 3.2% (FP) vs 2.5% (C) (P = NS)
Dutta et al[21]	1075	8 of 446 (1.8%)a	64 of 629 (10%)a	<.001	<1500 g All infants on IV fluids 6 mg/kg/d × 5 d (started at birth)
McCrossan et al[22]	64	0 of 102 (0%)a,d No Candida-related deaths	6 of 110 (5.5%)a 4 Candida-related deaths	.03	<1500 g For 3 wk in high-risk patients
Fluconazole Prophylaxis Versus Nystatin Prophylaxis					
Violaris et al[23]	80	2 of 38 (5.3%) FPa No Candida-related deaths	6 of 42 (14.3%) NPa 1 Candida-related death	RR 0.37, 95% CI (0.08–1.72)	<1500 g and ≤7 days old RCT, Excluded 44 patients because of hemodynamic instability or GI concerns. Oral fluconazole (4 mg/kg) vs oral nystatin (100,000 U/mL every 6 h)until full enteral feeds In NP group: 3 NEC, 1 SIP, 2 sepsis deaths (7.5%)

(continued on next page)

Table 1
(continued)

Nystatin Prophylaxis Studies

	N	ICI incidence: Nystatin	ICI incidence: Placebo (P) or controls (C)	P Value	Comments
Sims et al[24]	67	2 of 33 (6%)[a]	11 of 34 (32%) (P)[a]	.01	Intubated <1250 g 1 mL (100,000 IU) q8h until 1 week after extubation
Ozturk et al[25]	948	17 of 475 (3.6%)[e] NP started at <72 h 16 of 115 (13.9%)[e] NP colonization group (P ≤ .001)	131 of 358 (36%)(C)[e]	≤.001 ≤.001	3 groups: (1) NP started by 72 h of life, (2) NP started when colonization detected (mean 2 weeks), (3) no NP given. Data on <1500 g only. No effect for infants >1500 g 349 infants <1000 g and only 30 infants <750 g
Ganesan et al[26]	1055	13 of 525 (2.5%)[a] 6 Candida-related deaths	29 of 530 (5.5%) (C)[a] 14 Candida-related deaths	<.0001	<1500 g <33 wk (n = 1459; 4.1% vs 1.8%; P = .0008) 1 mL (100,000 IU) q6h until feeding tube removed Infants with peritonitis and NEC did not receive NP but were included in the analysis
Howell et al[27]	14,778	0.54%[c] 1.2%[c]	1.2% (C)[c] 2.7% (C)[c]	<.0001 <.0001	>1500 g: Decrease of 56% <1000 g: Decrease of 54% Comparative study of NICUs using NP vs no antifungal prophylaxis

Abbreviations: C, historical controls; CI, confidence interval; CVC, central venous catheter; FP, fluconazole prophylaxis; GI, gastrointestinal; IV, intravenous; NEC, necrotizing enterocolitis; NP, nystatin prophylaxis; NS, no statistically significant difference; P, placebo; RCT, randomized controlled trial; RR, relative risk; SIP, Spontaneous intestinal perforation.

[a] Bloodstream, Urine and CSF infections during FP.
[b] Only 91 of the 178 patients received FP. Bloodstream infection occurred in 2 of those 91 FP-treated patients.
[c] Bloodstream and CSF infections.
[d] 31 of 102 received FP.
[e] Bloodstream infections only.

Fluconazole Prophylaxis and Resistance

In studies of immunocompromised adults, fluconazole prophylaxis has been shown to be efficacious in preventing invasive fungal infection without emergence of azole resistance and is recommended for many high-risk patients.[32] Several neonatal studies have examined resistance closely during the 2 to 3-year study periods and have not reported significant changes in resistant isolates colonizing or causing infection during a course of prophylaxis in any patient.[7,8,11–23,28] Manzoni and colleagues[30] examined colonization and infection due to *C glabrata* and *C krusei* (species of *Candida* known for intrinsic azole resistance) over a 10-year period, 4 years before and 6 years after starting fluconazole prophylaxis. They found that the colonization rate (4%) and infection rate (1%) with these species stayed the same between the 2 time periods. Sarvikivi and colleagues[33] studied the use of fluconazole prophylaxis over a 12-year period in a NICU and found no *C albicans* bloodstream infections (BSIs) or resistance, no *C glabrata* or *C krusei* BSIs, and only 2 cases of fluconazole-resistant *C parapsilosis* BSIs. This and other studies have revealed a higher risk of emergence of resistance with higher (>6 mg/kg) and more frequent (daily) dosing of fluconazole.[7,11,31,33] Additional studies of minimal inhibitory concentration have demonstrated no significant resistance among fungal strains causing colonization or infection over 5-, 6-, and 11-year time periods in various NICUs.[7,11,18,31]

Fluconazole prophylaxis administered at 3 mg/kg IV twice weekly while IV access is required seems to be the most effective schedule in preventing ICI while minimizing risk of emergence of fungal resistance. To further limit pressure on the organism to develop resistance, in documented or suspected ICI cases a nonazole antifungal agent (amphotericin B) should be used for treatment.

Safety of Fluconazole Prophylaxis

In randomized trials, no significant adverse effects have been reported in infants treated with fluconazole prophylaxis compared with placebo patients. The incidence of bacterial infections and NEC have been similar between the treatment and placebo groups. In 4 randomized placebo-controlled trials, there were no significant differences in direct bilirubin or liver enzymes. One retrospective study with historic controls reported a higher incidence of cholestasis in patients receiving fluconazole, but there was no statistically significant difference between groups at discharge (6.7% vs 3.6%, $P = .54$).[13] In a subsequent study, Healy and colleagues[18] demonstrated that when controlling for other factors, fluconazole prophylaxis was not associated with cholestasis. Thirty-one percent of patients who received fluconazole prophylaxis developed cholestasis during hospitalization, and 66% had other predisposing conditions. Using multivariate logistic regression, NEC and increasing days of total parenteral nutrition, but not increasing fluconazole prophylactic doses, were significantly associated with the development of cholestasis.

Fluconazole and Mortality

In a meta-analysis of 3 randomized controlled trials (RCTs), 10% (34 of 319) of the fluconazole-treated infants developed an ICI or died compared with 25% (51 of 206) of placebo patients ($P<.001$).[34] Healy and colleagues[17,18] also demonstrated that by targeting fluconazole prophylaxis in infants with birth weight less than 1000 g, they were able to eliminate all *Candida*-related mortality in their NICU (from 0.1% to 0%, $P = .004$). Also, over a 4-year period, the incidence of ICI significantly decreased from 7% to 1.8% ($P = .003$) in infants with birth-weight less than 1000 g and 0.6% to 0.3% ($P = .05$) for all NICU patients. A systematic review of all trials of fluconazole prophylaxis in NICU patients demonstrated that fluconazole prophylaxis decreased the incidence of ICI in infants weighing less than 1000 g by 91% (OR 0.09; 95% CI, 0.04–0.24: $P = .0004$) and in infants weighing less than 1500 g by 85% (OR 0.15; 95% CI, 0.08–0.26; $P<.0001$).[29] All-cause mortality was 11% for the fluconazole-treated group compared with 16.3% for controls (OR 0.74; 95% CI, 0.58–0.95; $P = .017$). Candida-related mortality was virtually eliminated (OR 0.04; 95% CI, 0.01–0.31; $P = .006$).

Cost of Prevention Versus Cost of Candidal Infection

Invasive fungal infections in neonates bears high financial costs. Two recent case-control studies have examined the effect of ICI on cost of hospitalization and length of hospital stay.[2,6] For infants with birth weight less than1000 g, the mean increase in hospital costs due to ICI was $39,045 with no difference in length of stay. For infants with birth weight of 1000 g or greater, there was an increase of $122,302 with an additional length of stay of 16 days. It has been estimated that ICI in preterm infants leads to increased hospital costs of $30,000,000 per year in the United States.

Fluconazole prophylaxis is inexpensive. At a representative US institution, the pharmacy cost of a 4- to 6-week course (using twice-weekly dosing) is $144 to $216 per patient. The pharmacy cost of nystatin prophylaxis (using thrice-daily dosing for 4 to 6 weeks, $314 to $473) is approximately twice as high as IV fluconazole prophylaxis. A retrospective study by Uko and colleagues[16] examined the cost of fluconazole prophylaxis and reported a significant cost-benefit of $516,702 over 18 months in their NICU.

Nystatin Prophylaxis

Nystatin was the first antifungal agent studied in preterm infants and has been the subject of one randomized clinical trial and 3 retrospective or epidemiologic studies. Sims and colleagues[24] examined antifungal prophylaxis with nystatin in an RCT of 67 intubated infants with birth weight less than 1250 g, and found a decrease in fungal BSI and urinary tract infections. Ozturk and colleagues[25] in a quasi-randomized prospective study demonstrated that nystatin prophylaxis was significantly more effective in decreasing fungal BSI when started in the first 72 hours after birth (fungal BSI decreased from 36% to 3.6%) compared with screening for colonization, then instituting nystatin (fungal BSI only decreased to 14%). In a retrospective study of infants weighing less than 1500 g in the United Kingdom (n = 1055), nystatin prophylaxis decreased fungal BSI from 5.5% to 2.5% ($P<.0001$).[26] Nystatin prophylaxis was not given to infants with peritonitis or NEC. In a multicenter epidemiologic study comparing preterm infants who received nystatin prophylaxis with those who did not receive antifungal prophylaxis (1993–2006; Australia and New Zealand), oral nystatin prophylaxis was associated with a decrease in BSI or meningitis in infants with birth weight less than 1500 g (1.23% to 0.54%, $P<.0001$) and in infants with birth weight less than 1000 g (2.67% to 1.23%, $P<.0001$).[27]

Fluconazole Versus Nystatin Prophylaxis

Many questions regarding fluconazole and nystatin prophylaxis remain unanswered, and only one study has compared the 2 strategies (**Table 2**). An RCT of infants with less than 1500 g birth weight compared oral fluconazole to oral nystatin prophylaxis started in the first 7 days and continued until full enteral feedings were achieved.[23] ICI occurred in 2 of 38 (5.3%) fluconazole-treated infants compared with 6 of 42 (14.3%) nystatin-treated infants. All-cause mortality was zero in the fluconazole-treated group compared with 6 of 42 (7.5%) in the nystatin-treated group ($P = .03$). Of the 6 deaths in the nystatin group, 3 were from NEC; 1, from focal

Table 2
Comparison of antifungal prophylaxis agents: Fluconazole versus Nystatin

	Fluconazole	Nystatin
Effect on Colonization	Decreases CVC, skin, gastrointestinal, and respiratory colonization	Only decreases gastrointestinal colonization
Route of Administration	Given intravenously Can be given to all high-risk infants with IV access	Given enterally Cannot be given to infants not on enteral feeds, such as those with NEC, intestinal perforation, or ileus
Level of Evidence	Multiple RCTs demonstrating efficacy, even in extremely preterm infants (A-I) Efficacy and safety data in >4000 infants in 14 studies	Only one RCT in intubated infants <1250 g birth weight (A-II). Unknown number of infants of low gestational age, Underpowered for fungal BSIs, significant decrease in UTIs Retrospective and epidemiologic data from 3 other studies (B-II)
Efficacy	Approximately 90% decrease in ICI (blood, urine, CSF, or peritonitis) in ELBW (<1000 g) infants Candida-related mortality decreased by 96%	Retrospective studies with approximately 55% decrease in ICI in ELBWs
Resistance	No Candida albicans resistance (A-I) Rare nonalbicans resistance (B-II)	No data on resistance
Dosing	Twice-weekly dosing	3–4 times per day
Safety	Multiple studies in extremely preterm infants with no adverse side effects	Little data in extremely preterm infants <26 weeks gestation. Duration of prophylaxis not well-defined High osmolality and high sucrose content Unclear if safe in patients not tolerating enteral feedings May predispose to NEC (B-I) Safety data understudied/not reported on effect on NEC and bacterial infections
Approximate cost of 4-week course	$144	$314

See **Box 1** for description of levels of evidence.
Abbreviations: CVC, central venous catheter; UTI, urinary tract infection.

bowel perforation; and 2 were sepsis-related (including 1 *Candida*-related death). This study raised the question of safety of enteral nystatin for extremely preterm infants when they are not on full enteral feedings. Safety data (eg, bacterial infections and NEC) are lacking in most nystatin prophylaxis studies. The oral suspension of nystatin contains a high concentration of sucrose (50% by weight) and a very high osmolarity of 3002 mOsm/L.[35,36] Comparatively, oral fluconazole has an osmolarity of only 300 mOsm/L. Several reports describe an association of hyperosmolar oral medications and NEC in preterm infants.[37] It has also been suggested that the high concentration of sucrose in nystatin might alter the intestinal flora and facilitate bacterial translocation.

Aside from the aforementioned oral fluconazole study, all other fluconazole prophylaxis studies have used IV administration in the first weeks. In several studies, once patients achieved full enteral feedings, fluconazole administration was changed to enteral to complete 4 to 6 weeks of prophylaxis. As previously discussed, most infants are not colonized with yeast at birth or have low colony counts, which makes them good candidates for antifungal prophylaxis shortly after birth. Antifungal prophylaxis with parenteral fluconazole is effective in preventing colonization of the skin, gastrointestinal and respiratory tracts, and central venous catheter, and preventing dissemination to multisite colonization as well as eradicating colonization.[7–10] Enteral fluconazole is 90% absorbed compared with nonabsorbable nystatin. Therefore, nystatin will only prevent or reduce gastrointestinal fungal colonization, whereas enteral fluconazole may also prevent colonization at other sites. However, the absorption and pharmacokinetics of enteral fluconazole has not been adequately studied in preterm infants, and its impact on multisite colonization is uncertain. For this reason, the IV route is recommended for fluconazole prophylaxis in preterm infants requiring IV catheters.

The evidence favors IV fluconazole for antifungal prophylaxis (see **Tables 1** and **2**). There is A-I evidence for the recommendation for fluconazole prophylaxis. Comparatively, fluconazole prophylaxis has greater efficacy compared with nystatin prophylaxis (88% compared with 54%) and safety in infants weighing less than 1000 g; lower costs; twice-weekly compared to 3 times a day administration and ability to administer it to all high-risk infants weighing less than 1000 g, even in the face of gastrointestinal disease (eg, NEC, bowel perforation, ileus) or not feeding enterally, whereas nystatin prophylaxis can not be given with intestional diseases.

ALTERNATIVE APPROACHES TO PREVENTION OF ICI

Some NICUs do not routinely use fluconazole prophylaxis against fungal infections in high-risk patients. The debate surrounding prophylaxis include the following: (1) empiric therapy for suspected ICI would be efficacious; (2) infection control measures can reduce ICI incidence; (3) patients in NICUs with a very low ICI rate may not benefit from prophylaxis; and (4) concern for the emergence of azole resistance among fungal strains. While there is A-I evidence in favor of fluconazole prophylaxis, there are no RCTs for alternative approaches. The pros and cons of antifungal prophylaxis are summarized in **Table 3**.

IS EMPIRIC THERAPY BETTER THAN PROPHYLAXIS?

Some studies have suggested that empiric antifungal therapy when an infant has a sepsis evalution may lower mortality and improve outcomes in very low–birth-weight infants with fungal sepsis.[38,39] A retrospective study added empiric antifungal therapy with late-onset sepsis evaluations in critically ill neonates weighing less than 1500 g[39]

Table 3
Pros and cons of antifungal prophylaxis for ELBW infants

	Pros	Cons
Efficacy	• >80% efficacy for fluconazole prophylaxis in reducing ICI • >50% efficacy for nystatin prophylaxis • Infection, death, and neurodevelopmental impairment could be prevented even if rates are low (2% or less) • A unified approach, as with GBS prophylaxis, has the most benefit	• Rates vary by country and NICU
ICI mortality	• Multicenter data report >20% mortality in ELBWs (A-II)	• Some single-center studies report no mortality (B-II) • Empiric therapy could eliminate mortality (B-II) • Appropriate treatment of documented infections could eliminate mortality
Neurodevelopmental impairment in survivors	• 57% NDI in infants weighing <1000 g. (A-II) • Neither CVC removal nor empiric therapy improved NDI. (A-II)	• Optimal treatment with CVC removal or empiric therapy in all patients may improve outcomes (needs further study)
ICI rate	• 5%–10% in infants weighing <1000 g when all ICI (BSI, UTI, meningitis, peritonitis) included (A-II) • 20% for infants 23–24 weeks' gestation (A-II)	• Some NICUs report lower rates of 2%–3% in infants <1000 g using only BSI and meningitis (B-II)
Cost	• Fluconazole is inexpensive • ICI increases hospital costs (A-II) • >$500,000 decreased costs over 18 months in one NICU	• Some infection control measures are inexpensive (B-II)
Safety	• All RCTs showed safety with no increase in liver function tests and no adverse effects; >4100 infants from all FP studies	• One retrospective study reported increased cholestasis with FP, though no significant difference at discharge. • Possible concern with osmolarity of nystatin and NEC in extremely preterm infants.
Azole resistance	• RCTs have not demonstrated increased azole resistance • Amphotericin (or a non-azole) is used for treating suspected or documented ICI. This appropriately treats ICI if resistance would occur and places less azole pressure on fungi to become resistant if exposed to high dose fluconazole for treatment.	• Concern resistance may still occur over time
Alternative approaches	• Empiric therapy and infection control measures not subjected to RCTs and impact unknown	• Other approaches (empiric therapy, infection control measures) might be efficacious

See **Box 1** for description of levels of evidence.
Abbreviations: BSI, bloodstream infection; CVC, central venous catheter; FP, fluconazole prophylaxis; GA, gestational age; GBS, group B streptococci; ICI, Invasive *Candida* Infections; NDI, neurodevelopmental impairment; NNT number needed to treat; UTI, urinary tract infection.

with additional risk factors for ICI. Risk factors in this study included receipt of vanco-mycin and/or third-generation cephalosporin for 7 days and one or more of the following: total parenteral nutrition, mechanical ventilation, therapy with corticoste-roids or H2 blocking agents, or signs of mucocutaneous candidal infection, such as a rash or thrush. In this retrospective study *Candida*-related mortality occurred in 11 of 18 historic controls who did not receive empiric therapy compared with 0 of 6 patients who received empiric amphotericin therapy. Although empiric or prompt standardized treatment (including prompt removal of central vascular catheters) may reduce *Candida*-related deaths, neurodevelopmental impairment may still occur in the survivors, particularly those with birth weight less than 1000 g.[5] NICUs success-ful in infection prevention view infections as preventable and focus on prevention instead of early detection and treatment.

INFECTION CONTROL MEASURES TO PREVENT ICI
Prenatal Detection and Eradication of Maternal Vaginal Candidiasis

In pregnancies complicated by preterm labor, screening and treatment of vaginal candidiasis may be beneficial in preventing candidal colonization of the newborn.[40,41] This approach may also prevent development of congenital cutaneous candidiasis, which, if untreated, leads to invasive infection.[7,42–44]

Neonatal Medication and Feeding Stewardship

Three medication practices have been associated with an increased risk of ICI: use of broad-spectrum antibiotics (third- or fourth-generation cephalosporins or carbape-nems); use of gastric acid inhibitors (H2 blockers); and postnatal dexamethasone use.[5,45–48] Use of these medications should be restricted to documented gram-nega-tive infection, gastritis, and severe lung disease during the high-risk period for candidal infection in preterm infants when they require central venous catheters, parenteral nutrition, or endotracheal tubes, respectively. Establishing medication stewardship with guidelines in individual NICUs may further aid in reducing the rate of health care-associated infections, including ICI.[49]

Developing feeding protocols and promoting breast milk feedings may aid in the prevention of NEC, which is associated with a high rate of ICI.[50–52] Initiation of enteral feeding in the first 3 days of life in hemodynamically stable ELBW infants has been associated with lower rates of fungal infections, presumably by promoting the estab-lishment of a more favorable and diverse microbiome to prevent fungal proliferation and dissemination.[5]

A "Bundled" Approach to Central Venous Catheter Management for Prevention of ICI

Standardized protocols for insertion and management of central venous catheters, attention to sterile practices, hub and dressing care, and closed medication delivery systems may prevent central line-associated BSIs (CLABSIs), including candide-mia.[53–58] Aly and colleagues[53] reported significant reduction in all CLABSIs and elim-ination of candidal infection using a "bundled" approach. The central line bundle in this study included antifungal prophylaxis, in addition to line placement, and maintenance interventions.

Lactoferrin

In an RCT of bovine lactoferrin (bLF) or bLF plus probiotics in infants weighing less than 1500 g, the incidence of late-onset sepsis was significantly lower in the bLF and bLF plus probiotics groups (5.9% and 4.6%, respectively) than in placebo patients

(17.3%).[59] Subanalysis found that invasive fungal infections were also significantly less common with lactoferrin alone compared with placebo. Further studies are under way to determine the impact of lactoferrin and/or probiotics in preventing late-onset sepsis and NEC in preterm infants.

WHY USE FLUCONAZOLE PROPHYLAXIS IN NICUS WITH A LOW RATE OF ICI?

Studies examining candidal BSI in neonates report widely ranging incidence among centers and a decline in incidence over time. Data from the National Nosocomial Surveillance System Hospitals from 1995 to 2004 (132 NICUs and 130,523 neonates in the United States) indicated that for infants weighing less than 1000 g at birth, 50% of NICUs had fungal BSI rates of 7.5%, and 25% had rates higher than 13.5%.[3] However, there was considerable variation between NICUs with 10th and 90th percentiles of 3% and 23%. During a shorter time period (1998–2001), a smaller United States multicenter study reported similar rates of fungal BSI.[45] The rate of ICI is higher than the rate of candidemia, because the organism has a propensity to invade tissues rather than remaining in the vascular space. Studies reporting only BSI have been shown to underestimate the burden of ICI by approximately 4% in infants weighing less than 1000 g.[7,19] ELBW infants with signs of sepsis and positive cultures for *Candida* from urine, CSF, or peritoneal fluid, but not blood are at risk of *Candida*-related mortality and morbidity.[19,60] Even NICUs with low rates of ICI can reduce the incidence further through prophylaxis. In a study from New Zealand and Australia of almost 15,000 infants weighing less than 1500 g at birth, Howell and colleagues[27] showed the benefit of antifungal prophylaxis even in NICUs with a baseline ICI rate of less than 2%. Finally, group B streptococcus prevention is universally applied to reduce GBS neonatal sepsis from 1 per 1000 (0.1%) to 0.3 per 1000 (0.03%), and antifungal prophylaxis should follow suit for a much more common and fatal disease in infants with birth weight less than 1000 g. Elimination of ICIs in extremely preterm infants is an achievable goal through antifungal prophylaxis.

CONCERNS OVER SAFETY AND RESISTANCE

Single- and multicenter RCTs of fluconazole prophylaxis and meta-analyses of these studies have demonstrated safety without significant emergence of resistance in more

Table 4
Estimated annual impact of fluconazole prophylaxis in US ELBW infants, based on baseline rate of ICI

Baseline Rate	Estimated Number of ICIs Per Year	ICIs Prevented Per Year[a]	*Candida*-Related Deaths Prevented Per Year[b]	NDI Cases Prevented Per Year[c]
10%	3000	2400	360	437
5%	1500	1200	180	218
4%	1200	960	144	175
2%	600	480	72	87

Based on birth rate of 30,000 ELBWs per year in the United States from National Vital Statistics, Center of Disease Control and Prevention-CDC, 2007 (www.cdc.gov).
  Abbreviation: NDI, neurodevelopmental impairment.
  [a] 80% decrease in ICI.
  [b] Using attributable mortality of 15%.[2,5]
  [c] Using attributable NDI of 21% (57.2% in ICI vs 35.8% in non-ICI cases).[5]

Box 1
Strategies to reduce ICI morbidity and mortality in neonatal ICU patients (level of evidence)[a]

1. Use antifungal prophylaxis (IV fluconazole) while IV access is in use (central or peripheral) for infants with birth weight less than 1000 g and/or 27 weeks' gestational age or less (A-I).

   a. There is B-I and B-II evidence for antifungal prophylaxis with nystatin but limited data in infants <750 g and <26 weeks gestation. Since fluconazole prophylaxis has greater efficacy compared to nystatin, efficacy in the most immature patients, is less expensive, and can be given to infants not feeding, the evidence currently would favor fluconazole prophylaxis in preterm infants.

2. Start treatment of documented infections with appropriate antifungal dosing and prompt catheter removal for candidal BSI. (A-II).

3. Decrease broad-spectrum antibiotic use (B-II).

   Restrict third- and fourth-generation cephalosporins and carbapenems to treatment of proven gram-negative infections.

4. Decrease H2 blocker and proton-pump inhibitor use (B-II).

   Use only for proven gastritis, and restrict use to 3 days or until symptoms resolved.

5. Decrease postnatal dexamethasone use (B-II).

   Use only for severe lung disease.

[a] *US Public Health Service Grading System for ranking recommendations in clinical guidelines*: Strength of recommendation and levels of evidence.[62,63] A: good evidence; B: moderate evidence; C: poor evidence. I: at least one randomized clinical trial; II: at least one well-designed but nonrandomized trial; III: expert opinions based on experience or limited clinical reports.

---

than 11 years when targeted prophylaxis is used in high-risk preterm infants during the period of highest infection risk (while vascular catheters are in place). Continued surveillance of resistance is critically important as more centers adopt antifungal prophylaxis.

IMPACT OF ANTIFUNGAL PROPHYLAXIS

Table 4 summarizes the estimated impact if universal fluconazole prophylaxis were implemented for all ELBW infants in the United States. To maximize the effect and target the highest-risk period, antifungal prophylaxis should be started in the first 2 days of life and continued until IV access is no longer required. The need for vascular access correlates with the major risk factors for ICI: the central venous catheter, parenteral nutrition, gastrointestinal disease, and antibiotics. Twice-weekly IV low-dose (3 mg/kg) fluconazole seems to have the greatest efficacy and safety without emergence of resistance in preventing ICI in ELBW infants.

SUMMARY

ICI is a major problem for preterm infants. Strategies to reduce ICI and its morbidity and mortality in NICU patients are summarized in **Box 1**. Empiric antifungal treatment for suspected ICI and standardization of treatment regimens (appropriate dosing with prompt central catheter removal for documented candidal BSI) have been shown to decrease ICI mortality, but they may not reduce the risk of neurodevelopmental impairment and other morbidities associated with these infections. Infection control practices are likely to contribute to reducing the rate of ICI, but this has not yet been shown in prospective studies. This all favors prevention with fluconazole prophylaxis, which has been shown in multiple RCTs to reduce ICI without emergence of resistance and without adverse effects during long study periods. Just as antibiotic prophylaxis has been implemented for prevention of early-onset group B streptococcal infections, development of local, national, and international guidelines to prevent invasive, life-threatening candidal infections in the highest-risk NICU patients should be developed.[29,32,61] Antifungal prophylaxis administered to infants with birth weight less than 1000 g and/or 27 weeks' gestational age or less can reduce and potentially eliminate ICIs and *Candida*-related mortality.

REFERENCES

1. Johnsson H, Ewald U. The rate of candidaemia in preterm infants born at a gestational age of 23–28 weeks is inversely correlated to gestational age. Acta Paediatr 2004;93:954–8.
2. Zaoutis TE, Heydon K, Localio R, et al. Outcomes attributable to neonatal candidiasis. Clin Infect Dis 2007;44:1187–93.
3. Fridkin SK, Kaufman D, Edwards JR, et al. Changing incidence of Candida bloodstream infections among NICU patients in the United States: 1995–2004. Pediatrics 2006;117:1680–7.
4. Stoll BJ, Hansen NI, Adams-Chapman I, et al. Neurodevelopmental and growth impairment among extremely low-birth-weight infants with neonatal infection. JAMA 2004;292:2357–65.
5. Benjamin DK Jr, Stoll BJ, Fanaroff AA, et al. Neonatal candidiasis among extremely low birth weight infants: risk factors, mortality rates, and neurodevelopmental outcomes at 18 to 22 months. Pediatrics 2006;117:84–92.
6. Smith PB, Morgan J, Benjamin JD, et al. Excess costs of hospital care associated with neonatal candidemia. Pediatr Infect Dis J 2007;26:197–200.
7. Kaufman D, Boyle R, Hazen KC, et al. Fluconazole prophylaxis against fungal colonization and infection in preterm infants. N Engl J Med 2001;345:1660–6.
8. Manzoni P, Stolfi I, Pugni L, et al. A multicenter, randomized trial of prophylactic fluconazole in preterm neonates. N Engl J Med 2007;356:2483–95.
9. Manzoni P, Farina D, Galletto P, et al. Type and number of sites colonized by fungi and risk of progression to invasive fungal infection in preterm neonates in neonatal intensive care unit. J Perinat Med 2007;35:220–6.
10. Manzoni P, Farina D, Leonessa M, et al. Risk factors for progression to invasive fungal infection in preterm neonates with fungal colonization. Pediatrics 2006; 118:2359–64.
11. Kaufman D, Boyle R, Hazen KC, et al. Twice weekly fluconazole prophylaxis for prevention of invasive candida infection in high-risk infants of <1000 grams birth weight. J Pediatr 2005;147:172–9.
12. Kicklighter SD, Springer SC, Cox T, et al. Fluconazole for prophylaxis against candidal rectal colonization in the very low birth weight infant. Pediatrics 2001;107: 293–8.
13. Aghai ZH, Mudduluru M, Nakhla TA, et al. Fluconazole prophylaxis in extremely low birth weight infants: association with cholestasis. J Perinatol 2006;26:550–5.
14. Manzoni P, Arisio R, Mostert M, et al. Prophylactic fluconazole is effective in preventing fungal colonization and fungal systemic infections in preterm neonates: a single-center, 6-year, retrospective cohort study. Pediatrics 2006;117:e22–32.
15. Bertini G, Perugi S, Dani C, et al. Fluconazole prophylaxis prevents invasive fungal infection in high-risk, very low birth weight infants. J Pediatr 2005;147: 162–5.

16. Uko S, Soghier LM, Vega M, et al. Targeted short-term fluconazole prophylaxis among very low birth weight and extremely low birth weight infants. Pediatrics 2006;117:1243–52.
17. Healy CM, Baker CJ, Zaccaria E, et al. Impact of fluconazole prophylaxis on incidence and outcome of invasive candidiasis in a neonatal intensive care unit. J Pediatr 2005;147:166–71.
18. Healy CM, Campbell JR, Zaccaria E, et al. Fluconazole prophylaxis in extremely low birth weight neonates reduces invasive candidiasis mortality rates without emergence of fluconazole-resistant Candida species. Pediatrics 2008;121: 703–10.
19. Weitkamp JH, Ozdas A, Lafleur B, et al. Fluconazole prophylaxis for prevention of invasive fungal infections in targeted highest risk preterm infants limits drug exposure. J Perinatol 2008.
20. Aziz M, Patel AL, Losavio J, et al. Efficacy of fluconazole prophylaxis for prevention of invasive fungal infection in extremely low birth weight infants. Pediatr Infect Dis J 2010;29:352–6.
21. Dutta S, Murki S, Varma S, et al. Effects of cessation of a policy of neonatal fluconazole prophylaxis on fungal resurgence. Indian Pediatr 2005;42:1226–30.
22. McCrossan BA, McHenry E, O'Neill F, et al. Selective fluconazole prophylaxis in high-risk babies to reduce invasive fungal infection. Arch Dis Child Fetal Neonatal Ed 2007;92:F454–8.
23. Violaris K, Carbone T, Bateman D, et al. Comparison of fluconazole and nystatin oral suspensions for prophylaxis of systemic fungal infection in very low birth-weight infants. Am J Perinatol 2010;27:73–8.
24. Sims ME, Yoo Y, You H, et al. Prophylactic oral nystatin and fungal infections in very-low-birthweight infants. Am J Perinatol 1988;5:33–6.
25. Ozturk MA, Gunes T, Koklu E, et al. Oral nystatin prophylaxis to prevent invasive candidiasis in Neonatal Intensive Care Unit. Mycoses 2006;49:484–92.
26. Ganesan K, Harigopal S, Neal T, et al. Prophylactic oral nystatin for preterm babies under 33 weeks gestation decreases fungal colonisation and invasive fungaemia. Arch Dis Child Fetal Neonatal Ed 2009;94:F275–8.
27. Howell AJ, Isaacs D, Halliday R. Oral nystatin prophylaxis and neonatal fungal infections. Arch Dis Child Fetal Neonatal Ed 2009;94:F429–33 adc.
28. Parikh TB, Nanavati RN, Patankar CV, et al. Fluconazole prophylaxis against fungal colonization and invasive fungal infection in very low birth weight infants. Indian Pediatr 2007;44:830–7.
29. Kaufman DA. Fluconazole prophylaxis: can we eliminate invasive Candida infections in the neonatal ICU? Curr Opin Pediatr 2008;20:332–40.
30. Manzoni P, Leonessa M, Galletto P, et al. Routine use of fluconazole prophylaxis in a neonatal intensive care unit does not select natively fluconazole-resistant Candida subspecies. Pediatr Infect Dis J 2008;27:731–7.
31. Kaufman DA, Boyle R, Grossman LB, et al. Fluconazole prophylaxis dosing and the resistance patterns in preterm infants over a 11-year period [abstract]. Pediatric Academic Society Annual Meeting. Vancouver (Canada), May 1, 2010. E-PAS20101370.7.
32. Pappas PG, Kauffman CA, Andes D, et al. Clinical practice guidelines for the management of candidiasis: 2009 update by the Infectious Diseases Society of America. Clin Infect Dis 2009;48:503–35.
33. Sarvikivi E, Lyytikainen O, Soll DR, et al. Emergence of fluconazole resistance in a Candida parapsilosis strain that caused infections in a neonatal intensive care unit. J Clin Microbiol 2005;43:2729–35.

34. Kaufman D. Fluconazole prophylaxis decreases the combined outcome of invasive Candida infections or mortality in preterm infants. Pediatrics 2008;122: 1158–9.
35. Jew RK, Owen D, Kaufman D, et al. Osmolality of commonly used medications and formulas in the Neonatal Intensive Care Unit. Nutr Clin Pract 1997;12: 158–63.
36. Ernst JA, Williams JM, Glick MR, et al. Osmolality of substances used in the intensive care nursery. Pediatrics 1983;72:347–52.
37. Mutz AE, Obladen MW. Hyperosmolar oral medication and necrotizing enterocolitis. Pediatrics 1985;75:371–2.
38. Makhoul IR, Kassis I, Smolkin T, et al. Review of 49 neonates with acquired fungal sepsis: further characterization. Pediatrics 2001;107:61–6.
39. Procianoy RS, Eneas MV, Silveira RC. Empiric guidelines for treatment of Candida infection in high-risk neonates. Eur J Pediatr 2006;165:422–3.
40. Waggoner-Fountain LA, Walker MW, Hollis RJ, et al. Vertical and horizontal transmission of unique *Candida* species to premature newborns. Clin Infect Dis 1996; 22:803–8.
41. Freydiere AM, Piens MA, Andre JM, et al. Successful treatment of Candida glabrata peritonitis with fluconazole plus flucytosine in a premature infant following in vitro fertilization. Eur J Clin Microbiol Infect Dis 2005;24:704–5.
42. Baley JE, Kliegman RM, Boxerbaum B, et al. Fungal colonization in the very low birth weight infant. Pediatrics 1986;78:225–32.
43. Bliss JM, Basavegowda KP, Watson WJ, et al. Vertical and horizontal transmission of Candida albicans in very low birth weight infants using DNA fingerprinting techniques. Pediatr Infect Dis J 2008;27:231–5.
44. Kaufman DA. Neonatal candidiasis: clinical manifestations, management, and prevention strategies. J Pediatr 2010;156:s53–67.
45. Cotten CM, McDonald S, Stoll B, et al. The association of third-generation cephalosporin use and invasive candidiasis in extremely low birth-weight infants. Pediatrics 2006;118:717–22.
46. Benjamin DK Jr, DeLong ER, Steinbach WJ, et al. Empirical therapy for neonatal candidemia in very low birth weight infants. Pediatrics 2003;112:543–7.
47. Stoll BJ, Temprosa M, Tyson JE, et al. Dexamethasone therapy increases infection in very low birth weight infants. Pediatrics 1999;104:e63.
48. Watterberg KL, Gerdes JS, Cole CH, et al. Prophylaxis of early adrenal insufficiency to prevent bronchopulmonary dysplasia: a multicenter trial. Pediatrics 2004;114:1649–57.
49. Patel SJ, Oshodi A, Prasad P, et al. Antibiotic use in neonatal intensive care units and adherence with Centers for Disease Control and Prevention 12 step campaign to prevent antimicrobial resistance. Pediatr Infect Dis J 2009;28:1047–51.
50. Chapman RL, Faix RG. Persistently positive cultures and outcome in invasive neonatal candidiasis. Pediatr Infect Dis J 2000;19:822–7.
51. Uauy RD, Fanaroff AA, Korones SB, et al. Necrotizing enterocolitis in very low birth weight infants: biodemographic and clinical correlates. National Institute of Child Health and Human Development Neonatal Research Network. J Pediatr 1991;119:630–8.
52. Berseth CL, Bisquera JA, Paje VU. Prolonging small feeding volumes early in life decreases the incidence of necrotizing enterocolitis in very low birth weight infants. Pediatrics 2003;111:529–34.
53. Aly H, Herson V, Duncan A, et al. Is bloodstream infection preventable among premature infants? A tale of two cities. Pediatrics 2005;115:1513–8.

54. Curry S, Honeycutt M, Goins G, et al. Catheter-associated bloodstream infections in the NICU: getting to zero. Neonatal Netw 2009;28:151–5.
55. Schulman J, Wirtschafter DD, Kurtin P. Neonatal intensive care unit collaboration to decrease hospital-acquired bloodstream infections: from comparative performance reports to improvement networks. Pediatr Clin North Am 2009;56:865–92.
56. Schulman J, Stricof RL, Stevens TP, et al. Development of a statewide collaborative to decrease NICU central line-associated bloodstream infections. J Perinatol 2009;29:591–9.
57. Powers RJ, Wirtschafter DW. Decreasing central line associated bloodstream infection in neonatal intensive care. Clin Perinatol 2010;37:247–72.
58. Wirtschafter DD, Pettit J, Kurtin P, et al. A statewide quality improvement collaborative to reduce neonatal central line-associated blood stream infections. J Perinatol 2010;30:170–81.
59. Manzoni P, Rinaldi M, Cattani S, et al. Bovine lactoferrin supplementation for prevention of late-onset sepsis in very low-birth-weight neonates: a randomized trial. JAMA 2009;302:1421–8.
60. Benjamin DK, Stoll BJ, Goldberg R, et al. Neonatal candidiasis: epidemiology, clinical judgment, and outcomes [abstract]. Pediatric Academic Societies Annual Meeting. Honolulu (HI), May 2008. E-PAS 2008:633235.2.2008.
61. Candidiasis. In: Pickering L, Kimberlin DW, Baker CJ, et al, editors. Red book: 2009 report of the committee on infectious diseases. Elk Grove Villiage (IL): American Academy of Pediatrics; 2009. p. 245–9.
62. The periodic health examination. Canadian Task Force on the periodic health examination. Can Med Assoc J 1979;121:1193–254.
63. West S, King V, Carey TS, et al. Systems to rate the strength of scientific evidence. Evid Rep Technol Assess (Summ) 2002;1–11.

Strategies to Prevent Ventilator-Associated Pneumonia in Neonates

Jeffery S. Garland, MD, SM[a,b,c],*

KEYWORDS

- Ventilator-associated pneumonia
- Health care-associated infection • Neonate

Ventilator-associated pneumonia (VAP) is defined by the Centers for Disease Control and Prevention (CDC) as an episode of pneumonia in a patient who requires a device to assist or control respiration through a tracheostomy or endotracheal tube within 48 hours before the onset of the infection.[1] Health care-associated infections have a large impact on neonatal morbidity, survival, hospital costs, and length of stay.[2,3] VAP is a common cause and accounts for 6.8% to 32.2% of health care-acquired infections among neonates.[4–8] This article summarizes epidemiology, suspected pathogenesis, diagnosis, and strategies to prevent VAP in neonates.

EPIDEMIOLOGY

The exact rate of neonatal VAP is difficult to establish, because radiographic identification of pneumonia is difficult, especially among neonates with significant underlying lung disease, and diagnostic procedures commonly used in adults are rarely used in the neonatal intensive care unit (NICU). Differences in study methodology and case mix also influence the reported incidence of neonatal VAP.[9] National Nosocomial Infections Surveillance system data from 2004 showed that VAP rates for neonates weighing less than 1000 g ranged from 2.4 to 8.5 episodes per 1000 ventilator days.[10] In a cross-sectional study of 12 NICUs in children's hospitals, the incidence of VAP among neonates weighing less than 1000 g was 0 to 21.2 (median 3.5) per 1000 ventilator days.[11] Other investigators have reported rates varying from 12.5 to 52 infections per 1000 ventilator days.[4,12–16] Differences in study design and the case mix are likely responsible for the wide range of reported rates.

[a] Wheaton Franciscan Healthcare, St Joseph Hospital, Glendale, 5000 West Chamber, Milwaukee, WI 53210, USA
[b] Department of Pediatrics, Medical College of Wisconsin, 8701 West Watertown Plank Road, Milwaukee, WI 53226, USA
[c] Department of Pediatrics, University of Wisconsin School of Medicine and Public Health, 750 Highland Avenue, Milwaukee, WI, USA
* 3070 North 51 Street, Suite 309, Milwaukee, WI 53210.
E-mail address: jsgarland@hotmail.com

Clin Perinatol 37 (2010) 629–643
doi:10.1016/j.clp.2010.05.003
0095-5108/10/$ – see front matter © 2010 Elsevier Inc. All rights reserved.

perinatology.theclinics.com

Developmental abnormalities in the neonate's immune system including greater permeability of the skin and mucous membranes, decreased complement activity, and lower levels of immunoglobulins increase the susceptibility to health care-acquired infections. In a cohort of 742 neonates,[4] low birth weight (odds ratio [OR] 1.37; 95% confidence interval [CI], 1.01, 1.85] and mechanical ventilation (OR 9.7; 95% CI, 4.6, 20.4) increased pneumonia risk. Intravenous antibiotics were protective (OR 0.37; 95% CI, 0.21, 0.64). In another cohort of 229 ventilated neonates weighing 2000 g or less, VAP was more likely to occur in neonates who had a previous blood-stream infection (OR 3.5; 95% CI, 1.2, 10.8).[17] Organisms responsible for bloodstream infections were different from those causing VAP, suggesting that bloodstream infections may serve as a surrogate for severity of illness in the population. Although prolonged intubation before the episode of pneumonia did not reach statistical significance in this cohort, it was associated with VAP in the cohort reported by Yuan and colleagues.[12] Opiate treatment for sedation (OR 3.8; 95% CI, 1.8, 8.5), frequent endotracheal suctioning (OR 3.5; 95% CI 1.6, 7.4), and reintubation (OR 5.3; 95% CI, 2.0, 14.0) increased VAP risk in this study of ventilated neonates. Pneumonia is less common in neonates treated with nasal continuous positive airway pressure (NCPAP) when compared with those intubated on mechanical ventilation (12.5/1000 ventilator days vs 1.9/1000 NCPAP days, $P = .04$).[13] Finally, NICU design and staffing may affect VAP rates. Neonatal VAP decreased significantly when a NICU was moved from a crowded space to a larger unit with 50% more staffing.[18]

PATHOGENESIS

VAP occurs when bacterial, fungal, or viral pathogens enter the normally sterile lower respiratory tract and lung parenchyma. Under normal circumstances, anatomic barriers, cough reflexes, tracheobronchial secretions, mucociliary lining, cell-mediated and humoral immunity, and the phagocytic system of the alveolar macro-phages and neutrophils protect the lung parenchyma from infection. If these defenses are impaired, absent, or overcome by a high inoculum of organisms or those of unusual virulence, pneumonitis ensues.

Microorganisms responsible for VAP can originate from endogenous or exogenous sources (**Figs. 1** and **2**). Oropharyngeal or tracheobronchial colonization (endogenous source) with pathogenic bacteria begins with the adherence of microorganisms to the epithelial cells of the respiratory tract. Organisms causing VAP are often noted in the posterior pharynx.[19,20] Several investigators have highlighted[21–25] the role of pharyngeal and subglottic secretions in the development of VAP in adults. Contaminated oral and gastric secretions can pool above the cuff of the endotracheal tube in adult patients and gain access to the lower aspect of the respiratory tract by leaking around the cuff. Neonates are likely at greater risk for such aspiration of contaminated oral secretions, because endotracheal tubes used to ventilate neonates are not cuffed. Gram-positive organisms in the mouth colonize the trachea and endotracheal tubes within the first 48 hours of mechanical ventilation.[26,27] Gram-negative bacilli begin colonizing the endotracheal tube and trachea after 48 hours of respiratory support. VAP early after intubation tends to be more benign when compared with episodes that occur later in the hospital stay when gram-negative organisms begin to colonize the endotracheal tube.[27–29]

Support for the role of oropharyngeal colonization and subsequent tracheal colonization in the pathogenesis of VAP in neonates comes from studies showing a role of positioning in the acquisition of airway colonization with potential pathogens. Elevation of the head of the bed may reduce the risk of aspiration of contaminated

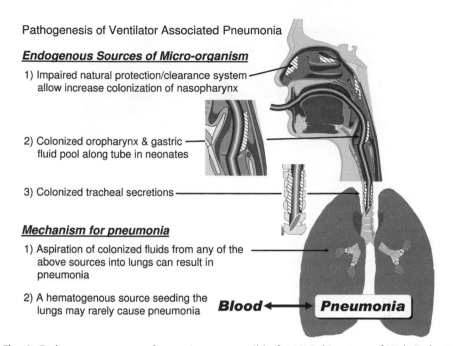

Pathogenesis of Ventilator Associated Pneumonia

Endogenous Sources of Micro-organism

1) Impaired natural protection/clearance system allow increase colonization of nasopharynx

2) Colonized oropharynx & gastric fluid pool along tube in neonates

3) Colonized tracheal secretions

Mechanism for pneumonia

1) Aspiration of colonized fluids from any of the above sources into lungs can result in pneumonia

2) A hematogenous source seeding the lungs may rarely cause pneumonia

Blood ↔ **_Pneumonia_**

Fig. 1. Endogenous sources of organisms responsible for VAP. (*Courtesy of* Walt Earhart, Wheaton Franciscan Healthcare; with permission. *Reproduced from* NeoreviewsPlus, copyright August 2010, Question 8, AAP; with permission.)

oropharyngeal and gastrointestinal contents in adults.[30] Aly and colleagues[31] reduced tracheal colonization from oropharyngeal contamination through lateral positioning of infants. Tracheal colonization was less common after 5 days of ventilation among neonates placed in a lateral position when compared with neonates nursed in a supine position (30% vs 87%, $P<.01$). The investigators speculate that by keeping the endotracheal tube and ventilator circuit in a horizontal position, secretions were less likely to track down from the oropharynx into the lower respiratory tract.

The stomach has been postulated as an additional reservoir for organisms responsible for VAP. The exact role gastric flora plays in the pathogenesis of VAP has been debated.[32,33] The contribution of gastric organisms to the pathogenesis of VAP is influenced by medications (antibiotics, antacids), supine head positioning, enteral feedings, and the patient's illness.[33,34] The position of a patient's body may reduce gastric reflux and subsequent tracheal aspiration and thus VAP risk. Torres and colleagues[35] demonstrated that technetium-labeled colloid inserted into a nasogastric tube was more likely to be noted in tracheal secretions of patients in a supine position than in those patients in a recumbent position. Drakulovic and colleagues[30] noted a higher rate of VAP in patients in a supine position when compared with patients in a semirecumbent position. Farhath and colleagues[36] noted that pepsin, a marker for gastric contents, was detected in the trachea of 92% of a cohort of ventilated neonates. The investigators did not evaluate associations between pepsin and VAP.

In summary, studies using rigorous culturing techniques have shown that oropharyngeal colonization plays a more important role in the development of endogenously acquired VAP than gastric colonization and subsequent aspiration.[27] Only rarely do organisms gain entry to the lower respiratory tract through blood or bacterial translocation from the gastrointestinal tract.

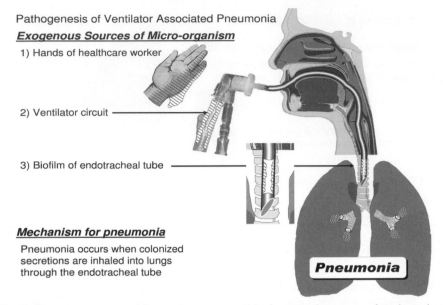

Fig. 2. Exogenous sources of organisms responsible for VAP. (*Courtesy of* Walt Earhart, Wheaton Franciscan Healthcare; with permission. *Reproduced from* NeoreviewsPlus, copyright August 2010, Question 8, AAP; with permission.)

Pathogens may also originate from exogenous sources (see **Fig. 2**). The endotracheal tube can serve as a reservoir for infecting microorganisms that adhere to the surface. Ventilator circuits, airway suctioning equipment, humidifiers, and nebulizers can become contaminated with pathogens that subsequently cause VAP.[19] Perhaps the most important source of exogenous contamination is from the caregivers' hands.[37] Gram-negative organisms, which begin colonizing the endotracheal tube later than gram-positive organisms, are frequently carried on the hands of caregivers.[38,39]

MICROBIOLOGY

Staphylococcus aureus and gram-negative organisms (*Pseudomonas aeruginosa, Eschericha coli, Klebsiella pneumoniae, Enterobacter* sp, and *Acinetobacter* sp) are the most common pathogens responsible for VAP in adults and pediatric patients. Apisarnthanarak and colleagues[17] noted gram-negative organisms in 94% of tracheal aspirates from neonates with VAP (**Table 1**). Multiple organisms were recovered from airway secretions in 58% of cases, and *S aureus* was recovered from approximately 25% of cases. Other investigators have also shown that neonatal VAP is mostly polymicrobial.[40] Webber and colleagues[40] cultured coliform species (44%), *P aeruginosa* (34%), and *S aureus* (15%) from the endotracheal tube or nasopharyngeal secretions of ventilated neonates with late-onset pneumonia. In a retrospective series examining risk factors for neonatal VAP,[12] more than 75% of the 28 VAP cases were due to gram-negative organisms (*K pneumoniae*, 39.3%; *P aeruginosa*, 25%; *Enterobacter cloacae* and *Citrobacter* sp, 3.6%). All studies evaluating the microbiology of neonatal VAP are limited by the fact that cultures are obtained from endotracheal aspirates and not from invasive sampling of the lower airway as in adults and thus may represent the oropharyngeal flora at the time of VAP.

Table 1
Organisms recovered from tracheal aspirates of 26 neonates with VAP[a]

Organism	Neonates with VAP (%)
Gram-Negative Rods	
P aeruginosa	38
Enterobacter spp	38
Klebsiella spp	23
E coli	15
Acinetobacter spp	8
Citrobacter spp	8
Stenotrophomonas maltophilia	4
Gram-Positive Cocci	
S aureus	23
Enterococcus	15
Group B Streptococcus	4

[a] VAP was considered to be present in infants receiving mechanical ventilation for at least 48 h who (1) developed new and persistent radiographic evidence of focal infiltrates at least 48 h after ventilation initiated and (2) received antibiotics for at least 7 days. Diagnosis of VAP confirmed by pediatric infectious disease fellow and neonatology attending. Because most infants had polymicrobial microorganisms, the sum of percentages is >100%.

Data from Apisarnthanarak A, Holzmann-Pazgal G, Hamvas A, et al. Ventilator-associated pneumonia in extremely preterm neonates in a neonatal intensive care unit: characteristics, risk factors, and outcomes. Pediatrics 2003;112:1286–9; with permission.

DIAGNOSIS AND TREATMENT

The major controversy regarding VAP in neonates is the criteria used to establish the diagnosis.[41] Stringent clinical criteria to define VAP have been developed by the CDC and the National Hospital Safety Network (NHSN). Criteria include mechanical ventilation within 48 hours of onset of suspected VAP; worsening gas exchange with an increase in oxygen or ventilatory requirements; 2 or more chest radiographs that show new infiltrates, consolidation, cavitation, or pneumatoceles; and at least 3 signs and symptoms. Signs and symptoms may include temperature instability, wheezing, tachypnea, cough, abnormal heart rate, change in secretions, or an abnormal leukocyte count. The problem with the criteria is the lack of a gold standard—microbiological identification of a pathogen from the lower respiratory tract, and thus the diagnostic value of the CDC surveillance recommendations is unknown.[41] The criteria have not been validated in neonates, and they are often open to subjective interpretation because they overlap with other diseases. Low-birth-weight neonates rarely develop cough, rhonchi, fever, or wheezing during an episode of pneumonia, and determining the presence of pneumonia from radiographs of low-birth-weight neonates with underlying chronic lung disease can be difficult.[14] Despite the difficulties with the CDC and NHSN criteria, they are still used to monitor VAP in NICUs and are frequently used by public and private reporting agencies.

Invasive testing is frequently used to diagnose pneumonia in ventilated adults with suspected VAP. Microbiologic examination of bronchoalveolar lavage (BAL) samples or those taken from a protected specimen brush (PBS) has an estimated 70% sensitivity and 77% specificity when compared with histopathology and/or lung tissue culture.[42–44] A meta-analysis of adult trials[45] determined that VAP could be confirmed with bronchoscopic samples in 44% to 69% of patients, and antibiotics were 3 times more likely to be changed when a bronchoscopy was done.

Bronchoscopy with lavage and PBS is not practical in neonates because of the size of the neonatal airway. Köksal and colleagues[46] used invasive testing with nonbronchoscopic BAL (NB-BAL) to obtain specimens from 145 ventilated neonates with suspected pneumonia. During the procedure, a 6F or 8F sterile catheter was passed through the endotracheal tube and wedged in the airway. About 90% of the 40 neonates with clinically diagnosed VAP had positive NB-BAL cultures. Sensitivity, specificity, positive predictive, and negative predictive values were 90%, 90%, 70%, and 97%, respectively. The percentage of intracellular bacteria in 2% or more of polymorphonuclear cells on Giemsa-stained smears was significantly higher in neonates with VAP when compared with colonized neonates (84% vs 26%, $P<.0001$). There were no significant complications. Although the results of Köksal and colleagues' study are intriguing, they are tempered by the fact that they were compared with clinically diagnosed VAP and not with a gold standard, such as a lung biopsy or tissue sample. Before accepting these results, the study should be replicated further to determine the diagnostic value and safety profile of the procedure.

Tracheal aspirate cultures and Gram stains are often included in the evaluation of neonates with suspected pneumonia. These tests have low sensitivity, specificity, and positive predictive value because it is difficult to distinguish between tracheal colonization and pneumonia.[47] In a retrospective cohort of neonates treated for VAP defined by clinical, radiographic, and tracheal aspirate results, 92% of cases had purulent tracheal aspirates (>25 leukocytes per high-power field); however, just 53% of cases had a positive tracheal culture.[12] In a cohort of very low-birth-weight infants, VAP, defined by the presence of clinical and radiographic findings as well as the presence of pathogens in the trachea or blood, was diagnosed in 5% of neonates without purulent aspirates and in just 10% of neonates with purulent aspirates.[48] When bacteria were not seen by Gram staining, purulence was noted in 11% of infants and 58% of infants had culture-positive tracheal aspirates. At the time of the first purulent tracheal aspirate, just 66% of neonates were symptomatic. The investigators did note that when a positive tracheal aspirate was associated with VAP, gram-negative organisms such as Klebsiella, Pseudomonas, and E coli were the most common isolates.[12,48] The predictive value of tracheal aspirates in ventilated adult patients is also limited.[49] Although tracheal aspirate findings have a low positive predictive value for pneumonia, they may play a role in helping to identify organisms colonizing the airway of infants at the time of a clinically diagnosed VAP. The knowledge of the sensitivities of the organisms colonizing the airway may help to guide antimicrobial choices, because the use of incorrect drugs has been associated with a significantly greater risk of death in adults with VAP.[50,51] A tracheal aspirate culture may also be of some value if it is negative in an adult patient who is either not on antibiotics or whose antibiotics have not been recently modified. In this instance, the negative predictive value is very high and the likelihood of pneumonia is close to zero.[52]

As with the diagnosis of VAP in neonates, there are no clear consensus guidelines for the optimal treatment of neonatal VAP. Based on adult trials, initial treatment should include broad empiric therapy. In selecting antimicrobial agents, likely flora and local resistance patterns should be considered. In most instances, a combination of several drugs is started. Initiating appropriate therapy has been shown to improve outcomes; however, the use of broad empiric coverage does carry the risk of increased resistance, toxicity, and cost. In adults, empiric monotherapy is recommended for uncomplicated VAP that is not likely due to a multidrug-resistant organism. Empiric combination therapy is recommended for more complicated disease. Adult treatment is tailored or discontinued based on culture results and clinical status. Because most neonates have multiple risk factors for multidrug resistance (such as prolonged mechanical ventilation, prior antibiotic exposure, multisystem illness) and there is no validated means of assessing VAP severity and improvement in neonates, most neonates with VAP usually receive a full course of empiric broad-spectrum antibiotics.

Empiric therapy usually includes an antipseudomonal agent such as piperacillin-tazobactam or ticarcillin-clavulanate that provides coverage for most gram-negative organisms and many gram-positive organisms. If local flora includes extended-spectrum β-lactamase producing organisms, carbapenems may be more appropriate for initial empiric therapy. The addition of another gram-negative agent such as an aminoglycoside is controversial. The addition of an aminoglycoside is appropriate if bacteremia is suspected or significant systemic symptoms are present. If the blood culture is negative and systemic symptoms are absent, de-escalating the therapy by discontinuing aminoglycosides is appropriate. Local epidemiology may dictate the use of dedicated gram-positive coverage for resistant organisms such as methicillin-resistant *Staphylococcus*. Depending on the quality and type of respiratory cultures, if no resistant organisms are detected, such therapy can be discontinued when the culture results are available.

PREVENTING VAP

The CDC[53] and American Thoracic Society[54] have published guidelines for the prevention of health care-associated pneumonia. Several studies have shown a reduction in VAP after the guidelines were implemented into a bundle of interventions that were implemented as a single intervention.[55–59] The power of the bundle is that it brings together several evidence-based practices that individually improve care but when applied together, may result in an even greater improvement in the desired outcome.

Most adult VAP prevention bundles recommend elevating the head of a ventilated patient's bed to between 30° and 45° to reduce the risk of aspiration of contaminated oropharyngeal and gastrointestinal contents. Drakulovic and colleagues[30] demonstrated that a semirecumbent position reduced the rate of clinically suspected (95% CI for difference, 10%–42%; P = .003) and microbiologically confirmed VAP (95% CI for difference, 4%–32%; P = .018). Only 1 underpowered pediatric trial presented in abstract form has evaluated this intervention and showed no effect. The results of Aly and colleagues'[31] and Farhath and colleagues'[36] studies suggest that using gravity may be an important means of preventing pathogens from gaining entry into the lower respiratory tract. However, Farhath and colleagues did not evaluate the association between the presence of pepsin in the trachea and VAP, and Aly and colleagues' work involved tracheal colonization and not pneumonia. Whether the best position to prevent VAP in ventilated neonates is the head of the bed kept up or a horizontal left or right lateral position of the neonate needs further study.

Because most organisms responsible for VAP originate from the oropharynx of ventilated patients, the CDC recommends that secretions be cleared from above the cuff of the endotracheal tube whenever the tube is repositioned or removed.[53] Although endotracheal neonatal tubes lack cuffs, the principle of suctioning out the oropharynx around the endotracheal tube before adjusting it or removing the tube could help reduce the risk of microaspiration of oropharyngeal secretions.

Introduction of closed multiuse suction catheters allowed endotracheal suctioning without disconnecting patients from the ventilator. Such closed suctioning methods reduce physiologic disruptions and arrhythmias, and nurses in the NICU judged such methods to be easier to use than an open suction system.[60] Closed suction systems present the potential for bacterial contamination when pooled secretions in the lumen are reintroduced into the lower respiratory tract with repeated suctioning. On the other hand, closed suctioning could potentially reduce environmental contamination of the endotracheal tube. Airway colonization is more common in ventilated adult patients suctioned with a closed system, but VAP rates have been reported to be equivalent[61,62] or slightly less than rates among patients with open system suctioning.[63] CDC recommendations do not endorse one system over the other, and there are no recommendations addressing the frequency at which closed suctioning systems should be changed.[53] In a study of 133 ventilated neonates randomized to a closed or open suction system, there were no differences in tracheal colonization patterns between groups nor in the VAP or bloodstream infection rates among treatment groups.

Breathing circuit condensate contamination can also serve as a mechanism for pathogenesis of VAP. The condensate that collects in the tubing should be drained away to prevent aspiration.[64] Breathing circuits do not need routine changing unless they become visibly soiled or malfunction.[53]

Most adult VAP reduction bundles recommend sedation vacations that allow a more accurate assessment of extubation readiness. In adults, the CDC recommends that the endotracheal tube be removed as soon as clinical indications allow and that noninvasive forms of respiratory support be used when feasible.[53] Because many centers use minimal or no sedation for ventilated neonates, actual use of sedation vacation is uncommon in most units. However, the process of assessing ventilated neonates on a daily basis to determine readiness for extubation should be built into the care team's daily rounds. The use of noninvasive measures such as NCPAP and nasal prong ventilation may help to reduce VAP rates. In time-sequenced cohort studies, reducing days of mechanical ventilation with either a high-flow nasal cannula or NCPAP decreased VAP incidence.[13,65] After extubation, repeat intubation should be avoided because of the increased risk of VAP associated with reintubation.[66]

Acidification of gastric contents decreases colonization with potential pathogens. Medications to prevent stress ulcer, such as H_2 antagonists and antacids that increase gastric pH, may increase gastric colonization and VAP risk. In 2 pediatric studies,[67,68] 1 retrospective and 1 prospective, there was no difference in VAP incidence among ventilated patients treated with sucralfate when compared with patients treated with agents that alter gastric pH. Pathogens responsible for VAP were similar across treatment groups. No studies have examined the associations between H_2 blockers and VAP among neonatal patients. However, necrotizing enterocolitis and gram-negative bacteremia have been associated with H_2 blocker use in neonates.[69,70] Current data do not support the use of peptic ulcer prophylaxis for the prevention of VAP among ventilated neonates.

Enteral nonabsorbable antimicrobials and topical antimicrobials applied to the oropharynx to decrease gastrointestinal colonization, better known as selective digestive tract decontamination (SDD), could potentially reduce respiratory tract infections caused by microaspiration of gastrointestinal organisms. Although several adult studies are supportive of SDD, CDC guidelines offer no recommendation for this procedure.[53] Studies of SDD to prevent VAP in ventilated children have conflicting results. In a randomized study of 226 ventilated patients in the pediatric intensive care unit,[71] those randomized to the SDD treatment group (colistin, tobramycin, and nystatin orally or through a nasogastric tube) had a lower frequency of pneumonia (2.6% vs 7.2%). Mortality was similar among treatment groups. In a small randomized trial (n = 23) of ventilated pediatric burn patients, there was no significant difference in VAP rates among controls and SDD-treated patients.[72] In a nonrandomized prospective trial of ventilated neonates, those who had SDD with administration of polymyxin E, tobramycin, and nystatin within the first 5 days of life had fewer nosocomial infections of intestinal origin.[73] VAP was not reported separately. Although SDD may have the potential for decreasing VAP risk, it could increase antibiotic resistance and certainly should be further evaluated before it is considered for neonates outside of clinical trials.

The CDC recommends a comprehensive oral hygiene program in patients at high risk for health care-associated pneumonia.[53] A meta-analysis by Pineda and colleagues[74] showed a reduction in VAP among adult patients treated by decontamination with oral

Table 2
Interventions often included in bundles to prevent VAP

Adult Interventions to Prevent VAP Not Applicable to Neonates	Adult or Pediatric Interventions to Prevent VAP Applicable to Neonates	Adult Interventions to Reduce VAP Unknown Risk: Benefit in Neonates
Cuffed endotracheal tubes (II[a])	Caregiver education (IA)	Elevation of head of the bed (II)
Subglottic suctioning of secretions (II)	Hand hygiene (IA)	Oral care with antiseptic solution (II)
Silver-coated endotracheal tubes	Wearing gloves when in contact with secretions (IB)	Orotracheal vs nasotracheal intubation (IB)
Deep venous thrombosis prophylaxis	Minimize days of ventilation (IB)	In-line (closed) suctioning
	Prevent gastric distension	Sedation vacation to assess extubation readiness
	Avoid unplanned extubation	Orogastric tube vs nasogastric tube
	Change ventilator circuit only when visibly soiled or malfunctioning (IA)	
	Disinfect respiratory equipment before storage (IA)	
	Remove condensate from ventilator circuit frequently (IB)	
	Avoid reintubation (II)	

CDC categorization of evidence-based recommendations.

Recommendations categorized based on existing scientific evidence, theoretic rationale, applicability, and potential economic impact in adult patients.

Category IA: Strongly recommended for implementation and supported by well-designed experimental, clinical, or epidemiologic studies.

Category IB: Strongly recommended for implementation and supported by certain clinical or epidemiologic studies and by strong theoretic rationale.

Category II: Suggested for implementation and supported by suggestive clinical or epidemiologic studies or strong theoretic rationale.

[a] Category of recommendation for adult patients.

chlorhexidine, although the reduction in VAP did not reach statistical significance. A meta-analysis by Chlebicki and Safdar[75] revealed a similar protective effect with chlorhexidine rinse. However, the CDC makes no recommendation for the use of an oral chlorhexidine rinse for the prevention of VAP in ill patients.[53] Chlorhexidine gluconate is not approved for neonates younger than 2 months, and there are little neonatal data to evaluate oral hygiene and VAP risk. It is likely that VAP pathogenesis differs in neonates who do not have gingivitis or the dental diseases of adults that would predispose them to abnormal oral colonization. Until further data are available, it seems prudent to follow the recommendation of the American Dental Association to wipe the gums and keep the mouth clean after feedings and when needed. Because oral suction equipment can become colonized with pathogens within 24 hours, separate suctioning equipment should be used for tracheal and oral secretions.

Reducing person-to-person transmission of bacteria is crucial to preventing nosocomial infections. Hand hygiene is likely the most important infection-control intervention in health care settings. Pathogens responsible for neonatal VAP are carried on the hands of health care workers and in the gastrointestinal tracts of infants. Respiratory equipments can become colonized with these organisms.[19] Thorough hand washing before and after contact with respiratory equipments should reduce cross-contamination between patients. In a time-sequence trial aimed at improving hand hygiene in the NICU, the rate of appropriate hand cleansing increased from 43% at baseline to 80% during the intervention period. The rate of respiratory infections decreased from 3.35 to 1.06 per 1000 patient days ($P = .002$).[76] However, the trial was not randomized and other clinical practices may have changed during the study period.

Changes in endotracheal tube design have decreased the incidence of VAP in adults. Aspiration of subglottic secretions through a hole in the dorsal aspect of endotracheal tubes above the inflated cuff decreased VAP rates in adults.[24,77,78] The CDC recommends the use of such tubes in ventilated adults.[53] Such tubes are not available for neonates. In a randomized trial, VAP was reduced by 35% in patients ventilated with a silver-coated endotracheal tube when compared with patients ventilated with a conventional tube.[79] The investigators suggest that the silver coating works to

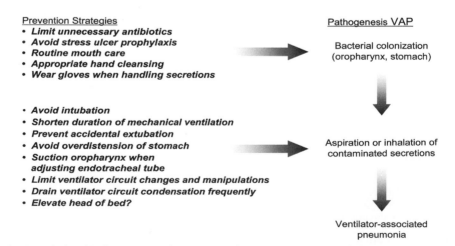

Fig. 3. Relationship between pathogenesis and strategies to prevent VAP.

prevent biofilm formation and bacterial colonization. Silver-coated endotracheal tubes are not available for neonates.

SUMMARY

Table 2 summarizes interventions that have been shown to effectively reduce VAP in adults and neonates. Potential interventions for inclusion in a neonatal VAP prevention bundle, which have not been evaluated in neonates but seem biologically plausible with good safety profiles, are also given. Fig. 3 summarizes how practical preventative interventions relate to the steps in the pathogenesis of VAP. Improved diagnostic criteria and surveillance techniques for VAP in the neonatal population need to be established before the effectiveness of these strategies can be accurately assessed.

ACKNOWLEDGMENTS

I would like to thank Mary O'Brien for her help with the preparation of the manuscript.

REFERENCES

1. Centers for Disease Control and Prevention. Criteria for defining nosocomial pneumonia. Available at: http://www.cdc.gov/ncidod/hip/NNIS/members/pneumonia/final/PneuCriteriaFinal.pdf. Accessed March 15, 2010.
2. Payne NR, Carpenter JH, Badger GJ, et al. Marginal increase in cost and excess length of stay associated with nosocomial blood stream infections in surviving very low birth weight infants. Pediatrics 2004;114:348–55.
3. Stoll BJ, Hansen NI, Adams-Chapman I, et al. Neurodevelopmental and growth impairment among extremely low birth weight infants with neonatal infection. JAMA 2004;292:2357–65.
4. van der Zwet WC, Kaiser AM, van Elburg RM, et al. Nosocomial infections in a Dutch neonatal intensive care unit: surveillance study with definitions for infection specifically adapted for neonates. J Hosp Infect 2005;61:300–11.
5. Gaynes RP, Edwards JR, Jarvis WR, et al. Nosocomial infections among neonates in high-risk nurseries in the United States. Pediatrics 1996;98:357–61.
6. Drews MB, Ludwig AC, Leititis JU, et al. Low birth weight and nosocomial infection of neonates in a neonatal intensive care unit. J Hosp Infect 1995;30:65–72.
7. Ford-Jones EL, Mindorff JM, Langley JM, et al. Epidemiologic study of 4684 hospital-acquired infections in pediatric patients. Pediatr Infect Dis J 1989;8:668–75.
8. Hemming VG, Overall JC, Britt MR. Nosocomial infections in a newborn intensive care unit. Results of forty-one months of surveillance. N Engl J Med 1976;10:1310–6.
9. Baltimore RS. Neonatal nosocomial infections. Semin Perinatol 1998;24:853–8.
10. CDC NNIS System. National Nosocomial Infections Surveillance (NNIS) system report, data summary from January 1992 through June 2004, issued October 2004. Am J Infect Control 2004;32:470–85.
11. Stover BH, Shulman DF, Bratcher M, et al. Nosocomial infection rates in US children's hospitals' neonatal and pediatric intensive care units. Am J Infect Control 2001;29:152–7.
12. Yuan TM, Chen LH, Yu H. Risk factors and outcomes for ventilator-associated pneumonia in neonatal intensive care unit patients. J Perinat Med 2007;35:334–8.

13. Hentschel J, Brüngger B, Stüdi K, et al. Prospective surveillance of nosocomial infections in a Swiss NICU: low risk of pneumonia on nasal continuous positive airway pressure. Infection 2005;33:350–5.
14. Cordero L, Ayers LW, Miller RR, et al. Surveillance of ventilator-associated pneumonia in very-low-birth-weight infants. Am J Infect Control 2002;30:32–9.
15. Pessoa-Silva CL, Richtmann R, Calil R, et al. Healthcare-associated infections among neonates in Brazil. Infect Control Hosp Epidemiol 2004;25:772–7.
16. Su BA, Hsieh HY, Chiu HY, et al. Nosocomial infection in a neonatal intensive care unit: a prospective study in Taiwan. Am J Infect Control 2007;35:190–4.
17. Apisarnthanarak A, Holzmann-Pazgal G, Hamvas A, et al. Ventilator-associated pneumonia in extremely preterm neonates in a neonatal intensive care unit: characteristics, risk factors, and outcomes. Pediatrics 2003;112:1283–9.
18. Goldmann DA, Freeman J, Durbin WA. Nosocomial infection and death in a neonatal intensive care unit. J Infect Dis 1983;147:635–41.
19. Sole ML, Poalillo FE, Byers JF, et al. Bacterial growth in secretions and on suctioning equipment of orally intubated patients: a pilot study. Am J Crit Care 2002;11:141–9.
20. Munro CL, Grap MJ. Oral health and care in the intensive care unit: state of the science. Am J Crit Care 2004;13:25–34.
21. Kollef M. The prevention of ventilator-associated pneumonia. N Engl J Med 1999;340:627–34.
22. de la Torre FJ, Pont T, Ferrer A, et al. Pattern of tracheal colonization during mechanical ventilation. Am J Respir Crit Care Med 1995;152:1028–33.
23. George DL, Falk PS, Wunderink RG, et al. Epidemiology of ventilator-acquired pneumonia based on protected bronchoscopic sampling. Am J Respir Crit Care Med 1998;158:1839–47.
24. Mahul P, Auboyer C, Jospe R, et al. Prevention of nosocomial pneumonia in intubated patients: respective role of mechanical subglottic secretions drainage and stress ulcer prophylaxis. Intensive Care Med 1992;18:20–5.
25. Valles J, Artigas A, Rello J, et al. Continuous aspiration of subglottic secretions in preventing ventilator-associated pneumonia. Ann Intern Med 1995;122:179–86.
26. Cendrero J, Solé-Violán J, Benítez A, et al. Role of different routes of tracheal colonization in the development of pneumonia in patients receiving mechanical ventilation. Chest 1999;116:462–70.
27. Feldman C, Kassel M, Cantrell J, et al. The presence and sequence of endotracheal tube colonization in patients undergoing mechanical ventilation. Eur Respir J 1999;13:546–51.
28. Hilbert G, Gruson D, Vargas F, et al. Noninvasive ventilation in immunosuppressed patients with pulmonary infiltrates, fever, and acute respiratory failure. N Engl J Med 2001;344:481–7.
29. Chastre J, Fagon J. Ventilator-associated pneumonia. Am J Respir Crit Care Med 2002;165:867–903.
30. Drakulovic MB, Torres A, Bauer TT, et al. Supine body position as a risk factor for nosocomial pneumonia in mechanically ventilated patients: a randomized trial. Lancet 1999;354:1851–8.
31. Aly H, Badawy M, El-Kholy A, et al. Randomized, controlled trial on tracheal colonization of ventilated infants: can gravity prevent ventilator-associated pneumonia? Pediatrics 2008;122:77–774.
32. Bonten MJ, Gaillard CA, van Tiel FH, et al. The stomach is not a source for colonization of the upper respiratory tract and pneumonia in ICU patients. Chest 1994;105:878–84.

33. Craven DE, Steger KA, Barber TW. Preventing nosocomial pneumonia: state of the art and perspectives for the 1990s. Am J Med 1991;91:445–535.
34. Kollef MH. Epidemiology and risk factors for nosocomial pneumonia. Emphasis on prevention. Clin Chest Med 1999;20:653–70.
35. Torres A, Serra-Batlles J, Ros E, et al. Pulmonary aspiration of gastric contents in patients receiving mechanical ventilation: the effect of body position. Ann Intern Med 1992;116:540–3.
36. Farhath S, He Z, Nakhla T, et al. Pepsin, a marker of gastric contents, is increased in tracheal aspirates from preterm infants who develop bronchopulmonary dysplasia. Pediatrics 2008;121:e253–9.
37. Alcón A, Fàbregas N, Torres A. Hospital-acquired pneumonia: etiologic considerations. Infect Dis Clin North Am 2003;17:679–95.
38. van Ogrot ML, van Zoeren-Grobben D, Verbakel-Salomons EM, et al. Serratia marcescens in infections in neonatal departments: description of an outbreak and review of the literature. J Hosp Infect 1997;36:95–103.
39. Szabó D, Filetoth Z, Szentandrassy J, et al. Molecular epidemiology of a cluster of cases due to Klebsiella pneumoniae producing SHV-5 extended-spectrum β-lactamase in the premature intensive care unit of a Hungarian hospital. J Clin Microbiol 1999;37:4167–9.
40. Webber S, Wilkinson AR, Lindsell D, et al. Neonatal pneumonia. Arch Dis Child 1990;65:207–11.
41. Baltimore RS. The difficulty of diagnosing ventilator-associated pneumonia. Pediatrics 2003;112:1420–1.
42. Chastre J, Viau F, Brun P, et al. Prospective evaluation of the protected specimen brush for diagnosis of pulmonary infections in ventilated patients. Am Rev Respir Dis 1984;130:924–9.
43. Fàbregas N, Ewig S, Torres A, et al. Clinical diagnosis of ventilator-associated pneumonia revisited: comparative validation using immediate postmortum lung biopsies. Thorax 1999;54:867–73.
44. Rouby JJ, Martin De Lassale E, Poete P, et al. Nosocomial bronchopneumonia in the critically ill. Histologic and bacteriologic aspects. Am Rev Respir Dis 1992; 146:1059–66.
45. Shorr AF, Sherner JH, Jackson WL, et al. Invasive approaches to the diagnosis of ventilator-associated pneumonia: a meta-analysis. Crit Care Med 2005;33:46–53.
46. Köksal N, Hacimustafaoğlul M, Celebi S, et al. Nonbronchoscopic bronchoalveolar lavage for diagnosing ventilator-associated pneumonia in newborns. Turk J Pediatr 2006;48:213–20.
47. Evans ME, Schaffner W, Federspiel CF, et al. Sensitivity, specificity and predictive value of body surface cultures in a neonatal intensive care unit. J Am Med Assoc 1988;259:248–52.
48. Cordero L, Sananes M, Dedhiya P, et al. Purulence and gram-negative bacilli in tracheal aspirates of mechanically ventilated very low birth weight infants. J Perinatol 2001;21:376–81.
49. Hill JD, Ratliff JL, Parrott JC, et al. Pulmonary pathology in acute respiratory insufficiency: lung biopsy as a diagnostic tool. J Thorac Cardiovasc Surg 1976;71:64–71.
50. Ibrahim EH, Sherman G, Ward S, et al. The influence of inadequate antimicrobial treatment of bloodstream infections on patient outcomes in the ICU setting. Chest 2000;118:146–55.
51. Chastre J, Luyt CE, Trouillet JL, et al. New diagnostic and prognostic markers of ventilator-associated pneumonia. Curr Opin Crit Care 2006;12:446–51.

52. Kirtland SH, Corley DE, Winterbauer RH, et al. The diagnosis of ventilator-associated pneumonia: a comparison of histologic, microbiologic, and clinical criteria. Chest 1997;112:445–7.

53. Centers for Disease Control and Prevention (CDC). Guidelines for prevention of healthcare-associated pneumonia. MMWR Recomm Rep 2004;53:1–36.

54. American Thoracic Society Infectious Diseases Society of America. Guidelines for the management of adults with hospital-acquired, ventilator-associated, and health care-associated pneumonia. Am J Respir Crit Care Med 2005;171:388–416.

55. Kollef MH. Prevention of hospital-associated pneumonia and ventilator-associated pneumonia. Crit Care Med 2004;32:1396–405.

56. Resar R, Pronovost P, Haraden C, et al. Using a bundle approach to improve ventilator care processes and reduce ventilator-associated pneumonia. Jt Comm J Qual Patient Saf 2005;31(5):243–8.

57. Lorente L, Blot S, Rello J. Evidence on measures for the prevention of ventilator-associated pneumonia. Eur Respir J 2007;30:1193–207.

58. Omrane R, Eid J, Perreault MM, et al. Impact of a protocol for prevention of ventilator-associated pneumonia. Ann Pharmacother 2007;41:1390–6.

59. Gastmeier P, Geffers C. Prevention of ventilator-associated pneumonia: analysis of studies published since 2004. J Hosp Infect 2007;67:1–8.

60. Cordero L, Sananes M, Ayers W. Comparison of a closed (Trach Care MAC) with open endotracheal suction system in small premature infants. J Perinatol 2000;3: 151–6.

61. Deppe SA, Kelly JW, Thoi LL, et al. Incidence of colonization, nosocomial pneumonia, and mortality in critically ill patients using a Trach Care closed-suction system versus an open-suction system: prospective, randomized study. Crit Care Med 1990;18:1389–93.

62. Johnson KL, Kearney PA, Johnson SB, et al. Closed versus open endotracheal suction: costs and physiologic consequences. Crit Care Med 1994;22:658–66.

63. Combes P, Fauvage B, Oleyer C. Nosocomial pneumonia in mechanically ventilated patients, a prospective randomized evaluation of the Stericath closed suctioning system. Intensive Care Med 2000;26:878–82.

64. Craven DE, Goularte TA, Make BJ. Contaminated condensate in mechanical ventilator circuits: a risk factor for nosocomial pneumonia? Am Rev Respir Dis 1984;129:625–8.

65. Holleman-Duray D, Kaupie D, Weiss MG. Heated humidified high-flow nasal cannula: use and a neonatal early extubation protocol. J Perinatol 2007;27: 776–81.

66. Torres A, Gatell JM, Aznar E, et al. Re-intubation increases the risk of nosocomial pneumonia in patients needing mechanical ventilation. Am J Respir Crit Care Med 1995;152:137–41.

67. Lopriore E, Markhorst D, Gemke R. Ventilator-associated pneumonia and upper airway colonization with Gram negative bacilli: the role of stress ulcer prophylaxis in children. Intensive Care Med 2002;28:763–7.

68. Yildizdas D, Yapicioglu H, Yilmaz H. Occurrence of ventilator-associated pneumonia in mechanically ventilated pediatric intensive care patients during stress ulcer prophylaxis with sucralfate, ranitidine, and omeprazole. J Crit Care 2002; 17:240–5.

69. Graham PL, Begg MD, Larson E, et al. Risk factors for late onset gram-negative sepsis in low birth weight infants hospitalized in the neonatal intensive care unit. Pediatr Infect Dis J 2006;25:113–7.

70. Guillet R, Stoll BJ, Cotten CM, et al. Association of H2-blocker therapy and higher incidence of necrotizing enterocolitis in very low birth weight infants. Pediatrics 2006;117:e137–42.
71. Ruza F, Alvarado F, Herruzo R, et al. Prevention of nosocomial infection in a pediatric intensive care unit (PICU) through the use of selective digestive decontamination. Eur J Epidemiol 1998;14:719–27.
72. Barret JP, Jeschke MG, Herndon DN. Selective decontamination of the digestive tract in severely burned pediatric patients. Burns 2001;27:439–45.
73. Herruzo-Cabrera R, Garcia Gonzalez JI, García-Magan P, et al. Nosocomial infection in a neonatal intensive care unit and its prevention with selective intestinal decolonization: a multivariant evaluation of infection reduction. Eur J Epidemiol 1994;10:573–80.
74. Pineda LA, Saliba RG, El Solh AA. Effect of oral decontamination with chlorhexidine on the incidence of nosocomial pneumonia: a meta-analysis. Crit Care 2006;10:R35.
75. Chlebicki MP, Safdar N. Topical chlorhexidine for prevention of ventilator-associated pneumonia: a meta-analysis. Crit Care Med 2007;35:595–602.
76. Won S, Chou H, Hsieh W, et al. Handwashing program for the prevention of nosocomial infections in a neonatal intensive care unit. Infect Control Hosp Epidemiol 2004;25:742–6.
77. Pneumatikos I, Koulouras V, Nathanail C, et al. Selective decontamination of subglottic area in mechanically ventilated patients with multiple trauma. Intensive Care Med 2002;28:432–7.
78. Kollef MH, Skubas NJ, Sundt TM. A randomized clinical trial of continuous aspiration of subglottic secretions in cardiac surgery patients. Chest 1999;116:1339–46.
79. Kollef MH, Afessa B, Anzueto A, et al. Silver-coated endotracheal tubes and incidence of ventilator-associated pneumonia: the NASCENT randomized trial. JAMA 2008;300(7):805–13.

Simple Strategies to Reduce Healthcare Associated Infections in the Neonatal Intensive Care Unit: Line, Tube, and Hand Hygiene

Philip L. Graham III, MD, MSc[a,b,c,*]

KEYWORDS

• Neonatal • Neonatal Intensive Care Unit
• Bloodstream infection • Urinary tract infection

Infants in the neonatal intensive care unit (NICU), particularly preterm infants, are among the most vulnerable patients at risk of developing healthcare associated infections (HAI). Risk factors for infections include the relative immunodeficiency of the neonate, frequent instrumentation, and need for invasive procedures performed during hospitalization.

In the past 50 years, the epidemiology of pathogens in NICUs has changed. In the 1950s, *Staphylococcus aureus* phage type 80/81 was the dominant hospital-acquired pathogen, whereas in the 1960s, *Pseudomonas aeruginosa*, *Klebsiella* spp, and *Escherichia coli* were most common.[1] In the 1970s, coagulase negative staphylococci (CONS) and methicillin-resistant *S aureus* (MRSA) became the most important causes of hospital-acquired infections in the NICU.[2] Today, with the advent of prepartum prophylaxis for high-risk deliveries, the incidence of early onset group B streptococcal infections has decreased substantially.[3]

The author has nothing to disclose.
[a] Division of Pediatric Infectious Diseases, Columbia University College of Physicians and Surgeons, New York, NY, USA
[b] Department of Pediatrics, Weill Cornell Medical College, 520 East 70th Street, New York, NY 10021, USA
[c] Department of Infection Prevention and Control, Division of Quality and Patient Safety, New York-Presbyterian Hospital, 520 East 70th Street, New York, NY 10021, USA
* 622 West 168th Street, PH4W-469, New York, NY 10032.
E-mail address: Pg143@columbia.edu

Clin Perinatol 37 (2010) 645–653
doi:10.1016/j.clp.2010.06.005
0095-5108/10/$ – see front matter © 2010 Elsevier Inc. All rights reserved.

gram-positive cocci continue to cause the largest proportion of late-onset infections, and many including MRSA, CONS, and vancomycin-resistant *Enterococcus faecium* (VREF) are multidrug resistant (MDR).[4–6] Gram-negative bacilli have also become increasingly MDR.[5,7] MDR gram-negatives elaborating several extended-spectrum β-lactamases (ESBL) and *Klebsiella pneumoniae* carbapenemases (KPCs) are of particular concern in the NICU given the lack of effective antibiotics. In addition, *Candida* species, particularly *Candida albicans* and *Candida parapsilosis*, have become increasingly common.[8]

In the past 2 decades, the number of infants hospitalized in NICUs has increased as a result of life-saving therapies and assisted reproduction technologies.[2] In the United States, approximately 12% of infants are born prematurely and approximately 40,000 have very low birthweight (<1500 g).[9,10] The incidence of HAI is inversely proportional to birthweight.[5–8,11] Clearly, effective strategies are needed to prevent infections in these patients.

Infections in the NICU are commonly related to device use and include central line–associated bloodstream infections (CLABSIs), ventilator-associated pneumonia (VAP), and catheter-associated urinary tract infections (CA-UTIs). Although primary prevention of these device-associated infections relies on minimizing their use, novel technologies such as antiseptic and antimicrobial impregnated catheters and meticulous care during their insertion and maintenance are key. Hand hygiene plays a significant part in the reduction of each of these types of infection. Additional benefits of hand hygiene include preventing the transmission of viral infections (eg, respiratory syncytial virus, adenovirus, influenza) and reducing the emergence of multidrug resistant organisms (MDROs) such as MRSA, VRE, ESBL-producing gram-negatives, and carbapemem-resistant gram-negatives.

HAND HYGIENE

Hand hygiene is the single most important strategy for avoiding transmission of contagions. In the NICU, flora is shared between patients and staff.[12,13] The gastrointestinal (GI) tract as well as the nares, nasopharynx, respiratory tract, and skin of colonized infants can serve as reservoirs for potential pathogens that are then spread patient-to-patient by transient or persistent carriage on health care providers' (HCP) hands.[12–14] Effective hand disinfection with an alcohol-containing degerming agent or an antimicrobial soap removes transient flora from the hands of HCPs. Although hand hygiene may seem simple, significant research has explored this issue and revealed complexities and obstacles. The guidelines for hand hygiene in health care settings published in the Centers for Disease Control's *Morbidity and Mortality Weekly Report* in 2002 offers important information and detailed advice, including variables that influence adherence to good hand hygiene. These variables are listed in adapted form in **Box 1**.[15]

Fingernails may also play a role in transmission of microorganisms. It has been demonstrated that artificial nails worn by HCPs are a risk factor for persistent hand carriage of potential pathogens including bacteria and fungi.[16–18] As a consequence, HCPs wearing artificial nails may be the cause of outbreaks in NICU patients. Outbreaks of *P aeruginosa* have been associated with persistent hand carriage as a result of fungal nail bed disease,[19] artificial nails, and long natural nails.[20] Similarly, an outbreak of ESBL-producing *K pneumoniae* was linked to an HCP wearing artificial nails,[15] and a history of wearing artificial nails was associated with an increased

---

Box 1
Factors influencing adherence to hand-hygiene practice

Observed risk factors for poor adherence to recommended hand-hygiene practices

- Physician status (rather than a nurse)
- Nursing assistant status (rather than a nurse)
- Male sex
- Working in an intensive care unit
- Working during the week (vs the weekend)
- Wearing gowns/gloves
- Automated sink
- Activities with high risk of cross-transmission
- High number of opportunities for hand hygiene per hour of patient care

Self-reported factors for poor adherence with hand hygiene

- Handwashing agents cause irritation and dryness
- Sinks are inconveniently located/shortage of sinks
- Lack of soap and paper towels
- Often too busy/insufficient time
- Understaffing/overcrowding
- Patients needs take priority
- Hand hygiene interferes with health care worker relationships with patients
- Low risk of acquiring infection from patients
- Wearing of gloves/beliefs that glove use obviates the need for hand hygiene
- Lack of knowledge of guidelines/protocols
- Not thinking about it/forgetfulness
- No role model from colleagues or superiors
- Skepticism regarding the value of hand hygiene
- Disagreement with the recommendations
- Lack of scientific information of definitive effect of improved hand hygiene on HAI rates

Additional perceived barriers to appropriate hand hygiene

- Lack of active participation in hand-hygiene promotion at individual or institutional level
- Lack of role model for hand hygiene
- Lack of institutional priority for hand hygiene
- Lack of administrative sanction of noncompliers/rewarding compliers
- Lack of institutional safety climate

Data from Pittet D. Improving compliance with hand hygiene in hospitals. Infect Control Hosp Epidemiol 2000;21:381–6.

---

risk of hand carriage of *P aeruginosa*.[19] As a result, the Hospital Infection Control Practices Advisory Committee (HICPAC) has crafted hand-hygiene guidelines that recommend that HCPs with direct patient contact should not be permitted to wear artificial nails.[15]

STRATEGIES TO PREVENT CLABSI

The Society for Healthcare Epidemiology of America (SHEA)/Infectious Diseases Society of America (IDSA)'s *Compendium of Strategies to Prevent Healthcare Associated Infections* provides detailed and evidence-based strategies to reduce device-related infections and other HAI.[21] In addition, several governmental, public health, and professional organizations have published evidence-based guidelines and/or implementation aids regarding the prevention of CLABSI. These organizations include: the Healthcare Infection Control Practices Advisory Committee,[22] the Institute for Healthcare Improvement,[23] and Making Health Care Safer, Agency for Healthcare Research and Quality.[24]

NICU patients have a high rate of CLABSIs compared with patients in other ICUs. The reasons for this include the relative immunodeficiency of low birthweight infants, frequent insertion of multiple catheters, repeated catheter access, and the need for catheter use for extended periods for prolonged nutritional support. In addition, some bloodstream infections in NICU patients may be misclassified when in fact bacterial translocation from an infant's GI tract is responsible for the infection. In these cases, the catheter is actually an innocent bystander rather than the cause of bacteremia.[10,25]

Reducing and eventually eliminating CLABSIs in the NICU requires a multimodal strategy. Infrastructure requirements include adequate numbers of nursing staff, infection prevention and control programs, information technology to collect and calculate catheter days as a denominator for computing rates of CLABSI and patient days to allow calculation of central venous catheter (CVC) use, resources to provide appropriate education and training, and adequate laboratory support for timely processing of specimens and reporting of results.

Practical implementation strategies include, but are not limited to, education of all HCPs about prevention of CLABSIs, development and implementation of a catheter insertion checklist, and education of HCPs about proper maintenance of catheter sterility.[15]

Catheter insertion kits and carts containing all necessary items for insertion are an integral part of a CLABSI reduction plan. Having all the necessary equipment and supplies in an easily accessible location aids in compliance with insertion guidelines. Maintaining such kits and carts can be an operational challenge, but should be a priority in NICUs because it may have a significant effect on reducing nosocomial infection rates.

Specific strategies to reduce CLABSIs may be divided into 3 time periods: before, during, and after CVC insertion. HCPs involved in the insertion, care, and maintenance of CVCs, and therefore CLABSI prevention, must be educated about the indications for catheter use, appropriate catheter insertion and maintenance techniques, and general infection prevention strategies.[21] Furthermore, HCPs must periodically have their skills and knowledge assessed.

Before CVC Insertion

Any HCP who inserts CVCs should undergo a credentialing process, as established by the individual health care institution, to ensure their competency before they independently insert a CVC. These processes often include a specific number of observed insertions before independent insertion.

During CVC Insertion

A catheter checklist should be used to ensure adherence to infection prevention practices at the time of CVC insertion.[21] CVC insertion should be observed by a nurse, physician, or other HCP who has received appropriate education to ensure that aseptic technique is maintained. These observing HCPs must be empowered to stop the procedure if breaches in aseptic technique are observed. Hand hygiene with an alcohol-based waterless product or a hand wash with antiseptic soap and water before catheter insertion or manipulation is essential.[15] Maximal sterile barrier precautions must be used during CVC insertion.[21] Such precautions include a mask, cap, sterile gown, and sterile gloves worn by all HCPs involved in the catheter insertion procedure. The patient should be covered with a large sterile drape during catheter insertion. This recommendation can be a challenge in neonates because of the need to monitor clinical status and maintain normothermia during the insertion.

The use of chlorhexidine gluconate (CHG)–based antiseptic for skin preparation before CVC insertion is a well-established best practice in patients older than 2 months of age.[21] CHG products are not approved by the US Food and Drug Administration for children younger than 2 months of age. Published recommendations suggest povidone iodine for children in this age group. However, many NICUs report using CHG in low birthweight infants without complications. One potential approach is to use CHG for all nonumbilical catheter insertions in infants more than 48 hours old (with or without an alcohol wipe afterwards) with close monitoring for potential adverse events such as skin irritation.

After CVC Insertion

Meticulous care of central catheters must continue after insertion. Catheter hubs, needleless connectors, and injection ports must be disinfected before accessing the catheter. A suggested infection control practice is to use a 15-second scrub the hub technique in which alcohol or chlorhexidine-alcohol pads are used with friction to disinfect the catheter hub each time the line is accessed.

In adolescents and adults with CVCs, changing transparent dressings and performing site care with CHG-based antiseptic every 5 to 7 days (or more frequently if the dressing is soiled, loose, or damp) is a proven best practice for reducing CLABSIs.[21] There are no studies of this practice in neonates, in whom the risk of catheter dislodgment or migration must be considered as a potential adverse event. Further studies are needed on the effect of CVC dressing changes on CLABSI rates in NICU patients.

A critical consideration in reducing CLABSIs is that nonessential CVCs must be removed promptly. On a daily basis there should be a structured assessment of each patient's need for continued intravascular central access. The Joint Commission on Accreditation of Healthcare Organizations (JCAHO) mandates that a daily HCP assessment of the continued need for every CVC is documented in the medical record.

Process measures are important for evaluating compliance with established guidelines for reducing NICU CLABSIs. Some examples include measurement of the percentage of CVC insertion procedures in which compliance with appropriate hand hygiene was observed, observation of the use of maximal sterile barrier precautions, measurement of the percentage of patients with a CVC for whom there is documentation of daily assessment, and measurement of compliance with cleaning of catheter hubs and injection ports before they are accessed.

SURVEILLANCE AND REPORTING OF NICU CLABSIS

Surveillance for CLABSIs is crucial for comparing rates among units and studying the effect of preventative interventions. All NICU staff should be regularly informed of the incidence of CLABSI in their unit. CLABSI rates should be measured and reported using the National Healthcare Safety Network definitions and benchmarks and reported as number of infections per 1000 catheter days. These data should be reported on a regular basis not only to the clinical units but also to the physician and nursing leaders and hospital administrators overseeing the units. CLABSI incidence should be compared with historical data for individual units and with national rates (ie, data from the National Healthcare Safety Network) and also, when possible, with benchmarking programs such as the Vermont Oxford Network.[26]

Accountability for CLABSIs is critically important, as shown by the involvement of hospital administrators and regulatory agencies in process improvement. Each hospital's chief executive officer and senior management are responsible for ensuring that the health care system supports an infection prevention and control program that effectively reduces the risk of CLABSI. This includes ensuring that an adequate number of trained personnel are assigned to the infection prevention and control program. Direct health care providers (including physicians, nurses, aides, and therapists) and ancillary personnel (such as housekeeping and equipment processing personnel) are responsible for ensuring that appropriate infection prevention and control practices are used at all times. These practices include use of hand hygiene, adhering to standard and expanded isolation precautions, cleaning and disinfecting equipment and the environment, using aseptic technique when inserting and caring for CVCs, applying maximal barrier precautions, and performing and documenting a daily assessment of the need for a CVC.

States and municipalities are increasingly requiring public reporting on rates of CLABSI and other HAIs, and more such reporting should be expected in the future. In addition, hospital reimbursement from insurance providers (or lack thereof) may be tied to these outcomes.

STRATEGIES TO PREVENT CA-UTIS

Urinary tract infection is the most common HAI, and most of these infections are attributable to indwelling urethral catheters. NICU patients are less likely than other ICU patients to have indwelling urinary catheters, but the problem of CA-UTI remains significant. Urinary tract infection is the most important adverse outcome of urinary catheter use, and urosepsis with bacteremia and severe illness may occur in neonates. Catheter use is also associated with negative outcomes other than infection, including nonbacterial urethral inflammation,[27] urethral strictures,[28] and mechanical trauma.

The National Healthcare Safety Network definition of symptomatic healthcare associated urinary tract infection[29] is commonly used for older patients, but can be difficult to apply to neonates. Localizing signs and symptoms may not be present or may not be recognized in neonates. The most common clinical presentation is fever with positive urine culture results, without other localized findings. However, given the high prevalence of bacteriuria in patients with an indwelling urinary catheter, this definition lacks specificity.

The Society for Healthcare Epidemiology of America/Infectious Diseases Society of America's *Compendium of Strategies to Prevent Healthcare Associated Infections* provides detailed and evidenced-based strategies to reduce device-related infections and other HAIs, including CA-UTIs.[26]

The duration of catheterization is the most important risk factor for development of infection.[30] Limiting catheter use and, when a catheter is indicated, minimizing the duration of use, are obvious primary strategies for CA-UTI prevention. As with vascular catheters, daily or even more frequent assessment of continued need for a urinary catheter should be a standard part of clinical decision making.

In patients who require urinary catheterization, several strategies have been identified to prevent CA-UTI. However, the existing published data are essentially all on adult patients and largely not applicable to the neonatal population. In adults, a randomized study reported that in-and-out catheterization was as effective as the use of an indwelling catheter for management of postoperative urinary retention[31]; the applicability of this finding to neonates is unknown and risks of trauma may be higher. Catheter materials such as silver alloy may decrease bacteriuria but have not been shown to decrease symptomatic infection or other undesirable outcomes in adults.[32–34] Those catheters are not currently manufactured for the neonatal population.

As with CLABSI prevention, education and training are paramount for CA-UTI prevention; HCP need to be educated about CA-UTI prevention, including alternatives to indwelling catheters and procedures for catheter insertion, management, and removal. Insertion of urinary catheters must only occur when necessary for patient care and catheters should be left in place only as long as indications persist. HCPs must practice hand hygiene immediately before insertion of the catheter and before and after any manipulation of the catheter site or apparatus. Aseptic technique and sterile equipment must be used for insertion. HCPs must use gloves, a drape, and sponges; a sterile or antiseptic solution for cleaning the urethral meatus; and a single-use packet of sterile lubricant jelly for insertion. Catheters should be maintained in a sterile, continuously closed drainage system.

Hospital administration has some accountability for CA-UTIs as described earlier for CLABSIs. Because the validity of the current Centers for Disease Control and Prevention/National Healthcare Safety Network definition of CA-UTI for comparison of facility-to-facility outcomes is not established, external reporting of CA-UTI rates is not currently recommended.

SUMMARY

Hand hygiene and a rigorous infection prevention program can prevent most CLABSIs and CA-UTIs in NICUs and thus can improve neonatal outcomes. Understanding that therapeutic interventions such as central vascular catheters and urinary catheters carry significant risk, much of which can be modified, will advance infection control as NICUs move forward toward elimination of device-associated infections.

REFERENCES

1. Bettelheim KA, Lennox-King SM. The acquisition of *Escherichia coli* by new-born babies. Infection 1976;4:174–9.
2. Gladstone IM, Ehrenkranz RA, Edberg SC, et al. A ten-year review of neonatal sepsis and comparison with the previous fifty-year experience. Pediatr Infect Dis J 1990;9:819–25.
3. Centers for Disease Control and Prevention (CDC). Decreasing incidence of perinatal Group B streptococcal disease–United States, 1993–1995. MMWR Morb Mortal Wkly Rep 1997;46:473–7.
4. Baltimore RS. Late, late-onset infections in the nursery. Yale J Biol Med 1988;61:501–6.
5. Gaynes RP, Edwards JR, Jarvis WR, et al. Nosocomial infections among neonates in high-risk nurseries in the United States. National Nosocomial Infections Surveillance System. Pediatrics 1996;98:357–61.

6. Stoll BJ, Gordon T, Korones SB, et al. Late-onset sepsis in very low birth weight neonates: a report from the National Institute of Child Health and Human Development Neonatal Research Network. J Pediatr 1996;129:63–71.
7. Sohn AH, Garrett DO, Sinkowitz-Cochran RL, et al. Prevalence of nosocomial infections in neonatal intensive care unit patients: results from the first national point-prevalence survey. J Pediatr 2001;139:821–7.
8. Saiman L, Ludington E, Pfaller M, et al. Risk factors for candidemia in Neonatal Intensive Care Unit patients. The National Epidemiology of Mycosis Survey study group. Pediatr Infect Dis J 2000;19:319–24.
9. Martin JA, Hamilton BE, Sutton PD, et al. Births: final data for 2006. In: National vital statistics reports, vol. 57. Hyattsville (MD): National Center for Health Statistics; 2009. no. 7.
10. The Vermont-Oxford Trials Network: very low birth weight outcomes for 1990. Investigators of the Vermont-Oxford Trials Network Database Project. Pediatrics 1993;91:540–5.
11. Zafar N, Wallace CM, Kieffer P, et al. Improving survival of vulnerable infants increases neonatal intensive care unit nosocomial infection rate. Arch Pediatr Adolesc Med 2001;155:1098–104.
12. Graham PL, Morel AS, Zhou J, et al. Epidemiology of methicillin-susceptible Staphylococcus aureus in the neonatal intensive care unit. Infect Control Hosp Epidemiol 2002;23:677–82.
13. Gupta A, Della-Latta P, Todd B, et al. Outbreak of extended-spectrum beta-lactamase-producing Klebsiella pneumoniae in a neonatal intensive care unit linked to artificial nails. Infect Control Hosp Epidemiol 2004;25:210–5.
14. Fryklund B, Tullus K, Berglund B, et al. Importance of the environment and the fecal flora of infants, nursing staff, and parents as sources of gram-negative bacteria colonizing newborns in three neonatal wards. Infection 1992;20:253–7.
15. Boyce JM, Pittet D. Guideline for hand hygiene in health care settings: recommendations of the Healthcare Infection Control Practices Advisory Committee and the HICPAC/SHEA/APIC/IDSA Hand Hygiene Task Force. Infect Control Hosp Epidemiol 2002;23:S3–40.
16. Pottinger J, Burns S, Manske C. Bacterial carriage by artificial versus natural nails. Am J Infect Control 1989;17:340–4.
17. Hedderwick SA, McNeil SA, Lyons MJ, et al. Pathogenic organisms associated with artificial fingernails worn by healthcare workers. Infect Control Hosp Epidemiol 2000;21:505–9.
18. Saiman L, Lerner A, Saal L, et al. Banning artificial nails from health care settings. Am J Infect Control 2002;30:252–4.
19. Foca M, Jakob K, Whittier S, et al. Endemic Pseudomonas aeruginosa infection in a neonatal intensive care unit. N Engl J Med 2000;343:695–700.
20. Moolenaar RL, Crutcher JM, San Joaquin VH, et al. A prolonged outbreak of Pseudomonas aeruginosa in a neonatal intensive care unit: did staff fingernails play a role in disease transmission? Infect Control Hosp Epidemiol 2000;21:80–5.
21. Marschall J, Mermel L, Classen D. Strategies to prevent central line–associated bloodstream infections in acute care hospitals. Infect Control Hosp Epidemiol 2008;29(S1):S22–30.
22. O'Grady NP, Alexander M, Dellinger EP, et al. Guidelines for the prevention of intravascular catheter related infections. MMWR Recomm Rep 2002;51(RR-10):1–29.
23. Institute for Healthcare Improvement. Available at: http://www.ihi.org/IHI/Topics/CriticalCare/IntensiveCare/Changes/ImplementtheCentralLineBundle.htm. Accessed June 4, 2010.

24. Saint S. Prevention of intravascular catheter-associated infections. In: Rockville (MD): Agency for Healthcare Research and Quality; 2001. Making health care safer: a critical analysis of patient safety practices. Evidence report/technology assessment, no. 43:E058. 163–83. Available at: http://www.ahrq.gov/qual/haify09.htm#addclabsi. Accessed June 4, 2010.

25. Smith A, Saiman L, Zhou J, et al. Concordance of gastrointestinal tract colonization and subsequent bloodstream infections with gram-negative bacilli in very low birthweight infants in the neonatal intensive care unit. Pediatr Infect Dis J. [Epub ahead of print]. Available at: http://journals.lww.com/pidj/toc/publishahead%20DOI%2010.1097/INF.0b013e3181e7884f%20Accessed%207/2/2010. Accessed July 2, 2010.

26. Lo E, Nicolle L, Classen D, et al. Strategies to prevent catheter-associated urinary tract infections in acute care hospitals. Infect Control Hosp Epidemiol 2008;29:S41–50.

27. Talja M, Korpela A, Jarvi K. Comparison of urethral reaction to full silicone, hydrogel coated and siliconized latex catheters. Br J Urol 1990;66:652–7.

28. Robertson GS, Everitt N, Burton PR, et al. Effect of catheter material on the incidence of urethral strictures. Br J Urol 1991;68:61–7.

29. Horan TC, Andrus M, Dudeck MA. CDC/NHSN surveillance definition of health care-associated infection and criteria for specific types of infections in the acute care setting. Am J Infect Control 2008;36:309–32.

30. Saint S, Chenowith CE. Biofilms and catheter associated urinary tract infections. Infect Dis Clin North Am 2003;17:411–32.

31. Lau H, Lam B. Management of postoperative urinary retention: a randomized trial of in-out versus overnight catheterization. ANZ J Surg 2004;74:658–61.

32. Johnson JR, Kuskowski MA, Wilt TJ. Systematic review: antimicrobial urinary catheters to prevent catheter-associated urinary tract infection in hospitalized patients. Ann Intern Med 2006;144:116–27.

33. Topal J, Conklin S, Camp K, et al. Prevention of nosocomial catheter-associated urinary tract infections through computerized feedback to physicians and a nurse-directed protocol. Am J Med Qual 2005;20:121–6.

34. Dumigan DG, Kohan CA, Reed CR, et al. Utilizing national nosocomial infection surveillance system date to improve urinary tract infection rates in three intensive-care units. Clin Perform Qual Health Care 1998;6:172–8.

Meningitis in Neonates: Bench to Bedside

Denis Grandgirard, PhD[a], Stephen L. Leib, MD[a,b],*

KEYWORDS

- Bacterial meningitis • Pneumococcus
- Pediatric • Experimental animal model

Bacterial meningitis (BM) is a life-threatening disease characterized by an acute purulent infection of the pia, the arachnoid, and the subarachnoid space.[1] The resulting inflammation also involves the brain parenchymal vessels (vasculitis), the inner ear, and the parenchyma itself. This intense inflammatory reaction is potentially fatal for the patient and contributes to the development of brain injury and the subsequent occurrence of persisting neurofunctional sequelae. BM is an important cause of morbidity and mortality worldwide, especially in neonates and children. *Streptococcus agalactiae* (GBS), gram negative bacilli (*Escherichia coli*, *Enterobacter* species, *Klebsiella pneumoniae*, *Citrobacter diversus*), and *Listeria monocytogenes* are more frequent in neonates;[2] while *Streptococcus pneumoniae*, *Neisseriae meningitis*, and *Hemophilus influenzae* type b (Hib) are the most frequent causes encountered during acute BM in young children and adults.[3–5] *L monocytogenes* preferentially affects pregnant women, mother and newborn, patients with compromised cell-mediated immunity, and patients more than 60 years old.[6] Introduction of vaccines, including the pneumococcal conjugate vaccine PCV7, the *N meningitis* tetravalent conjugate vaccines covering serogroups A, C, W-135, and Y, and the Hib vaccine will continue to change the epidemiology of meningitis.[7] For example, routine immunization in young infants with the Hib conjugate vaccine has virtually eradicated meningitis caused by this organism in high-income countries.[5] Emergence of disease caused

Financial disclosure and conflict of interest: The authors declare that they received unrestricted research grants from Cubist Pharmaceuticals and from Novartis Pharma. SLL is a member of the advisory boards of Cubist Phamaceuticals and Novartis Pharma.

Work presented herein was supported in part by grants from the Swiss National Science Foundation (310030-116257), and by the UBS Optimus Foundation.

[a] Neuro-Infectiology Laboratory, Institute for Infectious Diseases, University of Bern, Friedbuehlstrasse 51, Bern 3010, Switzerland

[b] Clinic for Infectious Diseases, University Hospital, Bern, Switzerland

* Corresponding author. Neuro-Infectiology Laboratory, Institute for Infectious Diseases, University of Bern, Friedbuehlstrasse 51, Bern 3010, Switzerland.

E-mail address: stephen.leib@ifik.unibe.ch

Clin Perinatol 37 (2010) 655–676
doi:10.1016/j.clp.2010.05.004
0095-5108/10/$ – see front matter © 2010 Elsevier Inc. All rights reserved.

by serotypes not included in the currently used vaccines has become a challenge and a focus of new vaccine development.[8]

Patients in countries with limited resources face a less favorable prognosis because of limited access to health care resources, underlying conditions (malnutrition, HIV-coinfection), and inefficient or nonexisting vaccination programs. The situation in the sub-Saharan meningitis belt of Africa is particularly concerning. Global estimates for the year 2000 reported an incidence of 31 per 100,000 for Hib meningitis in children under five years of age.[9] The mean worldwide case fatality rate (CFR) was 43%. In Africa, the incidence was 46 per 100,000 and the CFR jumped to an alarming 67%. Half of the fatal cases of Hib meningitis worldwide (78,300) occurred in Africa (34,600).[9] In a similar survey for pneumococcal meningitis in children less than five years of age, the global incidence rate was 17 per 100,000 (38 for Africa) and the CFR was 59% (73% for Africa). Worldwide, 65,000 young children died from pneumococcal meningitis and 31,700 of those deaths were in Africa.[10]

Among pediatric patients who survive meningitis, 20% to 50% have serious and permanent neurologic sequelae. The incidence of these neurologic sequelae among children has not significantly improved over the last decades.[11] A comparison of outcomes in two national prospective studies in England and Wales showed that the incidence of serious disabilities in patients surviving meningitis was similar from 1985 to 1987 (25.5%) compared with 1996 to 1997 (23.5%). In a study of 1,584 five-year-old children who survived meningitis during their first year of life, a 10-fold increase in the risk of moderate-to-severe disabilities compared with controls was demonstrated.[12] Similar results were obtained in a study that determined the prevalence of serious sequelae among a cohort of five-year old children who had had neonatal meningitis. At five years, 39 per 166 (23%) children with a history of neonatal BM had a serious disability, a 16-fold increase in risk of serious disability compared with matched controls.[13] Another study of 158 children, 7 and 12 years after BM, demonstrated that differences in intellectual, academic, and high-level cognitive function between survivors of BM and controls were maintained at the 7- and 12-year assessments.[14]

A younger age at illness is associated with a poorer efficiency in performing linguistic and executive functions, suggesting that the cerebral insult associated with meningitis has a greater impact on a developing brain.[15]

PATHOPHYSIOLOGY OF BM

Our understanding of the pathophysiology of BM in neonates is mostly based on observations of human cases and studies in experimental models. Various immature animal models of BM are used, including newborn rats,[16] infant rats,[17] infant mice,[18] and newborn pigs.[19] Models of BM in adult animals have used rats, mice, rabbits, and guinea pigs. Processes of bacterial invasion have been investigated using different routes of inoculation, including intraperitoneal,[20] subcutaneous,[21] intravenous, and intranasal.[22] To study the pathophysiologic processes after bacterial invasion of the central nervous system (CNS), direct intracerebroventricular or intracisternal injections of the pathogen is used and results in the development of meningitis in nearly 100% of inoculated animals. The successful establishment of experimental models of meningitis due to GBS,[17,23,24] L monocytogenes,[25–27] S pneumoniae,[28,29] H influenzae,[30] and E coli;[31] as well as, to a limited extent, N meningitis[32–34] has been reported. Based on the current knowledge on the pathophysiology of BM, the authors arbitrarily divided the processes leading to BM into three steps of the disease progression to more easily group them into mechanistic entities: colonization and invasion of the CNS; bacterial multiplication and CNS inflammation; and development of brain damage (**Fig. 1**).

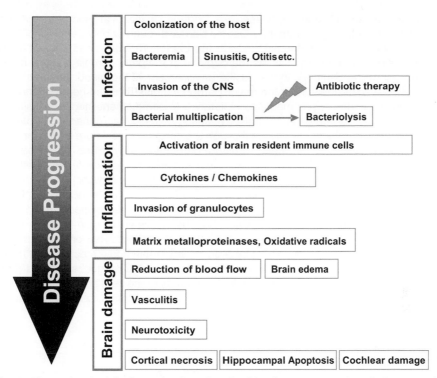

Fig. 1. The pathophysiologic mechanisms involved in disease progression during BM. The pathophysiology is arbitrarily divided into three phases. Prerequisite for infection beyond the immediate perinatal period is the colonization of the upper airways, and the process culminates with the virtually unhindered bacterial multiplication in the ventricular and subarachnoid spaces. Inflammation includes activation of the brain innate immune defense, the release of a cascade of inflammatory mediators and the recruitment of leukocytes. The development of brain damage results from combined effects of pathogen-derived factors and host factors, including deficits in brain perfusion and deleterious effects of inflammation.

Colonization and Invasion of the CNS

The majority of infections in neonates occur by vertical transmission, either in utero or during the passage through the birth canal. Meningitis in the newborn is often associated with sepsis. In young children and adults, colonization of the naso- or oropharynx or the sinuses by virulent strains is a prerequisite to the development of BM. Transmission usually occurs from person to person by the respiratory route, by large-droplet secretions. N meningitis is isolated in 10% to 35% of healthy adults,[35] but the vast majority of the strains are nonpathogenic.[36] Meningococcal carriage and acquisition are influenced by age, lifestyle, housing, close contact, and other factors.[37] The development of clinical infection usually occurs within 10 days or fewer after the acquisition of a pathogenic strain.[38] Marked variations in nasopharyngeal carriage of S pneumoniae and H influenzae have been reported between studies and geographic sites,[39] which have been related to genetic background and socioeconomic conditions such as housing, access to health care, hygiene, living conditions, and day care contact.

Colonization and invasion are also influenced by genetic determinants of the pathogen itself. Bacterial adhesins are required for optimal adhesion to the mucosal epithelium and specific endopeptidases are produced to inactivate secretory IgA anti-bodies. Bacteria then penetrate the mucosal barrier through or between the epithelial cells, depending on the pathogen.[40] Once the bacterium has gained access to the systemic circulation, the polysaccharide capsule of the pathogen plays a key role in the survival of the pathogen in the hostile environment of the blood. Encapsulation is therefore a shared feature of the major pathogens disseminated hematogenously. The polysaccharide capsule mediates resistance to complement-mediated lysis and phagocytosis by polymorphonuclear (PMN) leukocytes and macrophages. A potential route for bacteria entering the CNS is through the cerebral vasculature (blood-brain or blood-choroid barriers). Meningitis-causing pathogens may cross these barriers transcellularly or paracellularly. This traversal requires complex interplay between microbial factors and host receptors on the surface of brain microvascular endothelial cells. Endoplasmin, the 37 kDa laminin receptor, the platelet-activating factor receptor, and CD46 have all been described as receptors used by neurotropic path-ogens.[41] Alternatively, *L monocytogenes* has been shown to gain access to the CNS by transmigration of *L monocytogenes*-infected monocytes or myeloid cells across the blood-brain-barrier (BBB) by a so-called Trojan horse mechanism[42] or by retrograde axonal transport through cranial nerves.[43] Contiguous spread from mastoiditis, sinusitis or otitis; or a break in the integrity of the skull and meninges (mal-formations, trauma, and neurosurgery) have been demonstrated to be major causes for invasion by pneumococci.[44]

Bacterial Multiplication and CNS Inflammation

Once the CNS compartment is reached, the pathogen benefits from a much more favorable environment compared with the bloodstream. Host defense mechanisms are limited in the subarachnoid space by the anatomic blood brain barrier; there is minimal or no access to the cerebrospinal fluid (CSF) of complement factors, capsule-specific immunoglobulins, PMN leukocytes, and other plasma cells.[45] Subse-quently, bacteria multiply rapidly and spread unhindered over the entire surface of the brain and the spinal cord and into the Virchow-Robin space along the penetrating vessels (**Fig. 2**). Bacterial concentrations similar to those obtained in broth-culture in vitro (up to 10^9 colony-forming units per milliliter) can be reached. When the stationary growth phase is reached (in the case of pneumococci) or when bacteria are damaged by exposure to β-lactam antibiotics, they undergo bacteriolysis. The subsequent release of subcapsular bacterial components, including peptidoglycans, lipoteichoic acids, lipoproteins, lipopolysaccharides, bacterial DNA, or other cytosolic factors, are important triggers of the CNS inflammatory reaction. Immune sentinels that are able to recognize bacteria or bacterial components include active macro-phages and dendritic cells of the leptomeninges, the perivascular spaces, and the choroids plexus, as well as microglia cells of the brain parenchyma. Soluble or cellular signaling pattern-recognition receptors (PRRs) flag and recognize the pathogens and initiate the inflammatory cascade.[46] Typical PRRs, such as toll-like receptors (TLRs) and nucleotide-binding oligomerization domain proteins, have been shown to mediate the recognition of the pathogens in BM.[47,48] During pneumococcal meningitis, the combined activation of TLR2 and TLR4 leads to MyD88-dependent production of IL-1 family cytokines. These initial steps of immune recognition lead to the activation of many brain cells (ie, astrocytes, microglial cells, endothelial cells, ependymal cells, and resident macrophages) that produce early-response inflammatory cytokines such as IL-1β, tumor necrosis factor-α (TNF-α), and IL-6. These, in turn, trigger a cascade of inflammatory mediators, including other cytokines and chemokines, matrix-metalloproteinases (MMPs), and reactive oxygen species (ROS).[40,49] A profound

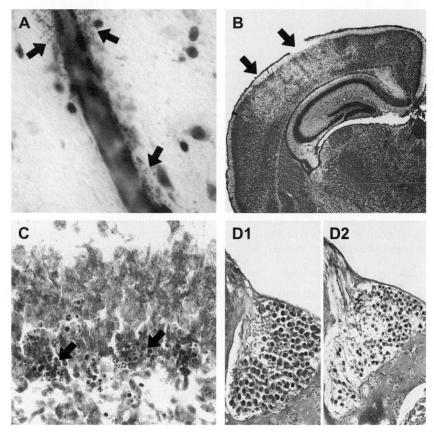

Fig. 2. Histomorphological features of neuronal damage in experimental pneumococcal meningitis in infant rats. (*A*) Subarachnoid space inflammation extending into the Virchow-Robin space consisting of bacteria (*arrows*) and inflammatory cells encircling the cortical vasculature. (*B*) Cortical injury in a wedge-shaped pattern suggestive of ischemic necrosis (*arrows*). (*C*) Hippocampal dentate gyrus histology in acute pneumococcal meningitis (36 hours after infection). Apoptotic cells (*arrows*) are characterized by fragmented nuclei forming round or oval so-called "apoptotic bodies" containing condensed chromatin materials. (*D1*) Spiral ganglion histology in an uninfected rat (control) and (*D2*) a littermate 3 weeks after BM. The marked reduction in neuronal density correlates with the extent of the hearing loss.

CSF pleocytosis in response to microbes invading the CNS is a characteristic feature of BM. The production of chemokines in the CSF establishes a chemotactic gradient necessary for the transmigration of leukocytes from the microvasculature to the site of inflammation. Chemokines are divided into the CXC chemokine family, which comprises those members in which the first two cysteines are separated by an intervening amino acid, and the CC family, where they are adjacent.[50] The Glu-Leu-Arg motif-containing (ELR+)-CXC and, to a lesser extent, CC chemokines are up-regulated during BM. In particular, the concentrations of IL-8[51] and CXCL5 in CSF[52] have been shown to correlate with the numbers of PMNs recruited to the CSF. Various factors released by PMNs, including cyto- and chemokines, oxidative radicals, and proteinases such as MMPs, have been shown to play a prominent role in the development of brain injury. MMPs have been shown to facilitate the extravasation of PMNs and to participate in BBB disruption by degrading components of the basal lamina of the cerebral vasculature.[53] CSF levels of MMP-9 in particular, were significantly higher in children who developed neurologic sequelae as a consequence of BM.[54] Acting as sheddases (membrane-bound enzymes that cleave extracellular portions of transmembrane proteins, releasing the soluble ectodomains from the cell surface) or convertases (enzymes that convert a compound into smaller, biologically-active compounds), MMPs participate in the production and the release of cytokines and their receptors. ROS and reactive nitrogen species are also produced by PMN and other immune competent cells within the CNS compartment. They lead to the production of peroxynitrite and the occurrence of membrane lipid peroxidation, as observed in inflammatory cells and penetrating cortical blood vessels in brain specimens from patients with meningitis[55] or during experimental pneumococcal meningitis in infant rats.[56] In addition, oxidants have been shown to induce DNA-strand breakage and subsequent poly (ADP-ribose) polymerase (PARP) activation, initiating an energy-consuming intracellular cycle that ultimately leads to cellular energy depletion and death, specifically in endothelial cells of the cerebral vasculature.[57,58]

Development of Brain Damage

The most frequent neurologic sequelae found in patients surviving meningitis include deafness, cerebral palsy, sensory-motor deficits, seizure disorders, and neuro-intellectual impairment, including deficits in learning and memory.[13,59] These neurofunctional consequences find their histomorphologic correlates in the tissue damage inflicted to the different structures of the brain during BM, including injury to the cortex, the hippocampus, and the inner ear (see **Fig. 2**).

Brain Injury to the Cortex

Focal sensorimotor deficits, seizure disorders, and cortical blindness result from cortical injury.[60] The cerebral vasculature plays a prominent role in the development of this type of injury. Microvascular injury through oxidative damage[56] and inflammatory alteration of the vessels (vasculitis) result in loss of cerebral vascular autoregulation, vasospasm, and reversible or permanent thrombosis. The cerebral vasculature of neonates is particularly susceptible to vasculitis.[61] Other factors that have shown to contribute to ischemic injury include the production of vasoconstrictive endothelins, the activation of platelets, and the induction of a procoagulant state.[62,63] Brain perfusion is further compromised by (1) an increase of the intracranial pressure brought about by brain edema due to cytotoxicity and breakdown of the BBB and (2) a decrease in systemic perfusion pressure due to bacteremia and the occurrence of sepsis syndrome. The synergy of these effects often results in cerebral ischemia and the development of cortical necrosis,[40] as found in autopsy cases[64] and animal models (see **Fig. 2**).[65]

Hippocampal Injury

In the hippocampus, apoptotic damage occurs in the subgranular zone (SGZ), the inner rim of the neuronal band within the dentate gyrus (see **Fig. 2**). This type of damage has been associated with learning and memory impairments in experimental models of pneumococcal meningitis[66-69] and likely represents the histomorphologic correlate of academic or behavioral limitations observed in survivors of neonatal and childhood BM. Activated caspase-3, an effector caspase responsible for executing the cell death program has been implicated in the molecular mechanism leading to hippocampal cell destruction during BM.[70,71] The vulnerable cells in the dentate gyrus include immature neurons recently generated from stem cells.[72,73] Stem or progenitor cells may also be targeted.[74]

A different form of hippocampal damage characterized by clusters of shrunken and pyknotic nuclei affects cells spanning the entire neuronal band of the dentate gyrus in newborn rats infected with GBS. This type of cell death is linked to the relocalization of the apoptosis-inducing factor to the nucleus.[75] A number of mediators have been proposed to act as molecular triggers for apoptosis in BM. Based on studies in animal models, brain cell death is mediated by components of the host inflammatory response including ROS, cytokines, and MMPs;[66] and by bacterial products such as pneumolysin and hydrogen peroxide from *S pneumoniae* and hemolysin from GBS.[76] Furthermore, an excessive release of glutamate has also been associated with the occurrence of hippocampal damage.[63,77] The mechanism by which bacteremia acts as an aggravating factor for hippocampal injury in experimental pneumococcal meningitis is undefined to date,[78] but may be linked to an increase in glial activation, the generation of nitric oxide and changes of Bax and Bcl-2 protein regulation critical for apoptosis, as demonstrated during systemic inflammation.[79]

The dentate gyrus, specifically the SGZ, is a site of a stem cell niche with continuous formation of new neurons.[80] Neurogenesis occurs lifelong in the SGZ of the dentate gyrus.[81,82] The hippocampus is therefore well-equipped for repair of damaged brain tissue. However, the capacity of self-repair is insufficient to compensate for the brain damage due to BM, as sequelae persist throughout childhood into adulthood.[14,15] Thus, the regenerative capacity of the hippocampus is likely to be permanently compromised by BM.[74] Subtle changes not detected on the anatomic level may occur, such as loss of a discrete cell subpopulation,[83] leading to cognitive or behavioral limitations.

Hearing Impairment

Hearing impairment following meningitis has been reported in 5% to 30% of patients, depending on the infecting pathogen.[44,84] Hearing loss characteristically develops at an early stage of BM.[85] In autopsy studies of patients who died from meningitis, infiltration of the temporal bones, by PMNs and eosinophils was found in the perilymphatic spaces, predominantly in the basal turn of the scala tympani. Hearing loss due to acute BM is related to damage of inner ear structures, including the blood-labyrinth barrier, hair cells, and spiral ganglion neurons.[86] In particular, the extent to which spiral ganglion neurons are reduced by BM correlates with the severity of permanent hearing loss (see **Fig. 2**).[87] Toxic effects of the pathogen (eg, pneumolysin or hydrogen peroxide for *S pneumoniae*), and host factors, including inflammatory mediators and ROS, appear responsible for the development of inner ear damage.[86]

STRATEGIES FOR PREVENTING NEURONAL DAMAGE DURING BM: CURRENT CONCEPTS

The current understanding of the pathophysiology of BM allows the identification of defined targets for therapies aimed at reducing the high mortality and the occurrence of neuronal damage (**Table1**).[88] These targets include:

Minimizing the release of bacterial components during bacterial killing
Inhibiting the production or the activity of inflammatory and neurotoxic mediators
Modulating the recruitment and the lifespan of invading PMN
Modulating apoptotic pathways
Ameliorating cerebral perfusion.

Table 1
Effects of pharmacologic interventions in experimental models of productive BM assessed by histopathological and functional outcome measurements

Pathomechanism	Intervention	Host Species	Pathogen	Cortical Damage	Hippocampal Apoptosis	Learning Capacity	Hearing Loss	References
Ischemia (vasoconstriction)	Endothelin antagonist (bosentan)	Infant rat	SP	↓	↔	—	—	Pfister et al[62]
Reactive oxygen species	PBN (radical scavenger)	Infant rat	SP	↓	↑	→	—	Loeffler et al[68]
		Infant rat	GBS	↓	↓[a]	→	—	Leib et al[17]
	NAC	Infant rat	SP	↓	↔	—	—	Auer et al[101]
		Adult rat	SP	—	—	—	→	Klein et al[102]
	MnTBAP, uric acid	Adult rat	SP	—	—	—	→	Klein et al, [102] Kastenbauer et al[147]
	DFO	Infant rat	SP	↓	↔	—	—	Auer et al[101]
	TLM	Infant rat	SP	↓	↔	—	—	Auer et al[101]
Nitric oxide	iNOS inhibition (aminoguanidine)	Infant rat	GBS	↑	—	—	—	Leib et al[24]
Matrix-metalloproteinases	GM6001 (MMP inhibitor)	Infant rat	SP	↓	—	—	—	Leib et al[148]
	BB-1101 (MMP & TACE inhibitor)	Infant rat	SP	↓	→	↑	—	Leib et al[66]
	TNF484 (MMP & TACE inhibitor)	Infant rat	SP	↓	↔	—	—	Meli et al[99]
	Doxycycline	Infant rat	SP	↓	↔	—	→	Meli et al[100]
TNF-α neutralization	Anti-TNF-Antibody	Infant rat	GBS	↔	↓[a]	—	—	Bogdan et al[149]
Attenuation of inflammation	Dexamethasone	Infant rat	SP	—	↑	→	↔	Leib et al[67], Coimbra et al[131]
	Dexamethasone	Adult rat	GBS	↓	—	↑	—	Irazuzta et al[130]
	Dexamethasone	Adult rat	SP	—	—	—	↔	Worsoe et al[132]
	Dexamethasone	Gerbils	SP	—	—	—	→	Addison et al[133]
	Dexamethasone	Rabbit	SP	—	—	—	→	Rappaport et al[134]

Category	Intervention	Animal	Pathogen				Reference
Neutrophils	Roscovitine	Adult mice	SP	→	—	—	Koedel et al[109]
	Fucoidin	Adult rat	SP	↔	—	—	Brandt et al[106]
Caspases	Caspase-3 inhibition (Ac-DEVD-CHO)	Infant rat	SP	—	→	—	Gianinazzi et al[70]
	Pan-caspase inhibition (Z-VAD-fmk)	Rabbit	SP	—	→	—	Braun et al[112]
Neurotrophin	BDNF	Infant rat	SP	—	→	—	Bifrare et al[113]
		Infant rat	GBS	→	→	—	Bifrare et al[113]
		Young rat	SP	—	—	→	Li et al[115]
Excitotoxicity	Kynurenic acid	Infant rat	GBS	→	→	—	Leib et al[23]
	Dextromethorphan	Infant rat	SP	↔	←	—	Sellner et al[150]
	RO 25-6981	Infant rat	SP	—	↔	—	Kolarova et al[151]
Antibiotic-induced bacterial wall release	Daptomycin	Infant rat	SP	→	↔	—	Grandgirard et al[65]
	Rifampicin	Rabbit	SP	—	→	—	Gerber et al,[93] Spreer et al[94]
	Clindamycin	Rabbit	SP	—	→	—	Bottcher et al[95]

Abbreviations: BDNF, brain-derived neurotrophic factor; DFO, deferoxamine; DG, dentate gyrus; MnTBAP, Mn(III)tetrakis-(4 benzoic-acid)-porphyrin); NAC, N-acetylcysteine; PBN, phenyl-(alpha)-tert-butyl-nitrone; SP, *S pneumoniae*; TLM, tirilazad mesylate.

a Damage in the DG consisting of pyknotic cells, distinct from caspase-dependent apoptosis.

Data from Refs.63,86,88,146

Minimizing the Release of Bacterial Components During Bacterial Killing

An important aspect with respect to outcome is to shorten the time from the first symptoms of BM to the initiation of antibiotic therapy.[89] Current guidelines recommend empiric therapy with β-lactam antibiotics that are rapidly bacteriolytic and thereby induce a brisk release of subcapsular bacterial components. Although antibiotic therapy reduces the overall release of bacterial components, when compared with unhindered replication and subsequent autolysis, the initial release of bacterial components has been shown to accentuate CSF inflammation.[90,91]

The use of antibiotics acting by inhibition of RNA-protein synthesis or DNA replication (rifamycins, macrolides, clindamycin, ketolides, and quinolones) reduces bacterial lysis.[92] In experimental disease models, rifampicin, given as a pretreatment, either 6 hours or 30 minutes before the initiation of therapy with ceftriaxone, reduced the release of bacterial components into the CSF and attenuated neuronal injury in the hippocampus.[93,94] Similarly, clindamycin was shown to lower extracellular concentration of hydroxyl radicals and glutamate, and to decrease neuronal apoptosis in the dentate gyrus in a rabbit model of pneumococcal meningitis.[95] The cyclic lipopeptide daptomycin kills bacteria by inducing a rapid depolarization of the bacterial membrane, shutting down the cellular metabolism without subsequent bacteriolysis, thus minimizing the associated release of bacterial components in experimental pneumococcal meningitis.[96] The use of daptomycin versus ceftriaxone resulted in less CSF inflammation and less brain damage.[29,65] As the antibacterial activity of daptomycin is limited to gram-positive pathogens, the clinical use of this antibiotic for empiric therapy of BM would require the combination with a broad spectrum antibiotic. In a recent study in rabbits with meningitis, the combination of daptomycin with ceftriaxone was shown to be more effective than vancomycin plus ceftriaxone.[97] A preclinical study of infant rats with pneumococcal meningitis showed that the combination of daptomycin with ceftriaxone led to less brain injury and attenuated hearing loss when compared with ceftriaxone or to the combination of ceftriaxone with rifampin.[98]

Inhibiting the Production or Activity of Inflammatory and Neurotoxic Mediators

A number of strategies have been evaluated in experimental models of BM, which, until now, have not been translated into clinical use (see **Table 1**). A major challenge seems to be the difficulty in identifying therapies that attenuate damage to the hippocampus, the cortex, and the inner ear. Experimental therapies using inhibitors of MMPs are generally protective against cortical damage. MMP-inhibition combined with TNF-α–converting enzyme (TACE) inhibitory activity has been shown to ameliorate cortical necrosis and limit apoptosis in the hippocampal dentate gyrus.[66] However, the beneficial effect on both forms of injury by an MMP/TACE inhibitor was restricted to one compound and could not be shown for other similar MMP/TACE inhibitors.[99] Thus the beneficial effect of MMP/TACE inhibition may not solely depend on the TACE inhibitory activity. Inhibiting MMPs by adjuvant therapy with doxycycline reduced the occurrence of cortical damage and attenuated hearing loss, but had no significant effect on hippocampal apoptosis.[100] Antioxidant therapies have been shown to protect from damage to the neocortex and the inner ear, but not from hippocampal apoptosis (see **Table 1**).[17,101–103] The antioxidant phenyl-{alpha}-tert-butyl-nitrone (PBN), although neuroprotective for the cortex, aggravated hippocampal apoptosis in experimental pneumococcal meningitis.[68] Adjuvant therapy with melatonin, which also has some antioxidant properties, had anti-inflammatory effects but did not reduce neuronal injury in a rabbit model of either gram-positive *S pneumoniae* or gram-negative *E coli* meningitis.[104]

Modulating the Recruitment and the Lifespan of Invading PMNs

Inhibiting leucocyte entry into the CSF to decrease the local inflammatory reaction would seem to be an attractive strategy during BM. Treatment with the polysaccharide fucoidin, a selectin blocker that inhibits leukocyte recruitment in the CSF, resulted in reduced CSF levels of IL-1β and, to a lesser extent, TNF-α during experimental pneumococcal meningitis.[105] However, a higher mortality was observed, with no measurable affect on brain damage or bacterial numbers in the CSF compartment.[106] Furthermore, leucocyte blockade affected the host's ability to control systemic infection, as demonstrated by an increase number of bacteria in the blood. An augmented peripheral neutrophil response by pretreatment with granulocyte-colony-stimulating factor reduced mortality and prevented brain damage with a concomitant decrease in blood and CSF bacterial titers.[107] However, an adverse effect on hearing loss was observed.[108] A more promising strategy to limit the detrimental effects of PMNs is controlling their lifespan rather than blocking their entry into the CNS.[109] This novel therapeutic approach is based on the observation that an enhanced lifespan of activated PMN in the CSF substantially contributed to massive leukocyte accumulation and meningitis-induced tissue injury. Roscovitin, a cyclin-dependent kinase inhibitor that induces caspase-dependent apoptosis in PMNs,[110] reduced CSF pleocytosis and led to less brain histopathology, better performance in clinical rating scales, and a lower mortality rate in experimental pneumococcal meningitis.

Modulating Apoptotic Pathways

Caspases are a family of cysteinyl-aspartate-directed proteases that cleave a wide range of cellular proteins, orchestrating morphologic changes (eg, the formation of apoptotic bodies, see **Fig. 2**) and signaling cascades during inflammatory and apoptotic processes.[111] Caspase inhibitors have been shown to attenuate hippocampal apoptosis in the dentate gyrus. The pan-caspase inhibitor z-VAD-fmk induced a down-modulation of inflammation and an associated inhibition of caspases,[112] whereas specific inhibition of caspase-3 with Ac-DEVD-CHO relied solely on the interference with the apoptotic pathway.[70]

Administration of exogenous brain-derived neurotrophic factor (BDNF) has been shown to attenuate all forms of brain damage associated with pneumococcal and with GBS meningitis.[113] Although the mechanism of action is still poorly understood, BDNF has been shown to beneficially modulate caspase-dependent and -independent pathways of neuronal damage and to improve neurofunctional outcome. The therapeutic strategy to administer exogenous BDNF has been further supported by the finding that antibiotic treatment decreased expression of endogenous BDNF in experimental pneumococcal meningitis.[114] BDNF has been shown to exert a protective effect on hearing capacity in experimental pneumococcal meningitis.[115]

Erythropoietin (EPO) treatment has been show to exert neuroprotective effect in different experimental paradigms.[116] By inducing the expression of prosurvival factors, such as Bcl-xL in the hippocampus,[117] one could reasonably expect that EPO treatment would reduce apoptosis in the hippocampus during BM. However, no beneficial effect upon EPO treatment could be observed in a rabbit experimental model of E coli meningitis.[118]

Preserving Cerebral Perfusion

The neuroprotective effect of antioxidants in the cortex may be attributed to an effect on the cerebral vasculature leading to amelioration of cerebral perfusion.[56]

Treatments with superoxide dismutase, catalase, or peroxinitrite scavengers such as uric acid, or Mn(III)tetrakis-(4 benzoic-acid)-porphyrin; as well as with other free radical scavengers such as N-acetyl cysteine (NAC) result in a reduction of intracranial pressure increase, edema formation, and CSF pleocytosis.[119–123] Modulation of nitric oxide synthase and nitric oxide production is potentially deleterious in BM as experimental studies suggest a disease-phase-dependent role at the level of cerebral vasculature.[124] Early in the disease, a vasodilatative effect of nitric oxide contributes to hyperemia; whereas later, when cerebral blood flow progressively declines, nitric oxide (produced by the vasculature) has a protective against ischemia and subsequent cortical necrosis.[24] Endothelins are potent vasoconstrictory peptides and CSF levels are increased in patients with BM.[125] Endothelin antagonists may have therapeutic potential by reducing cerebral vasoconstriction. In experimental meningitis, treatment with the endothelin antagonist bosentan prevented the reduction in cerebral blood flow and reduced the extent of cerebral ischemia.[62] The use of nonsteroidal anti-inflammatory drugs such as indomethacin has been shown to reduce brain edema, but had no effect on intracranial pressure.[126] Matrix metalloproteinase inhibition may have therapeutic potential, by preventing degradation of the endothelial basement membrane of the BBB,[53] thus limiting vasogenic edema and perfusion deficits.

UNPROVEN BENEFIT OF ADJUNCTIVE THERAPY WITH DEXAMETHASONE

Given the contribution of excessive inflammation to the development of brain damage in BM, treatment with dexamethasone has been recommended as adjunctive therapy. However, recent clinical and experimental studies do not universally support these recommendations.[67,127,128]

In an infant rat model of pneumococcal meningitis,[67] and in a rabbit model of E coli meningitis, dexamethasone treatment was shown to increase hippocampal injury.[129] In contrast, decreased neurologic sequelae and caspase activity were found in an adult rat model.[130] For hearing loss, conflicting results were also found in different experimental models—showing no significant benefit for pneumococcal meningitis in the infant rat;[131] protection of spiral ganglion neurons but no improvement of hearing capacity through intratympanic instillation in adult rats;[132] and, finally, an otoprotective effect in gerbils[133] and rabbits.[134] In children, the effect of adjuvant dexamethasone in the treatment of BM was evaluated in a number of studies and meta-analyses, with contradicting conclusions. For Hib meningitis, but not pneumococcal meningitis, a beneficial effect was found for hearing loss.[135] In a large placebo-controlled, double-blind, randomized trial including 598 children in resource-poor countries,[136] no difference in survival or neurologic sequelae could be found with addition of dexamethasone therapy. In a more recent study, the only significant effect of dexamethasone was to prevent deafness in children with Hib meningitis, without considering timing between dexamethasone and ceftriaxone administration.[128] This finding was challenged by results from another recent study, in which dexamethasone failed to prevent hearing loss regardless of the causative agent or the timing of antimicrobial agent.[137] A difference between low- and high-income countries regarding the efficacy of dexamethasone therapy was suggested in a recent meta-analysis, which found the use of corticosteroid therapy was beneficial only for adult patients in high-income countries.[138] The latest—and most complete—meta-analysis was performed by pooling the original data of five previously published meta-analyses. This analysis concluded that there was no effect of adjunctive dexamethasone for all or any subgroup of patients with BM.[127]

GLYCEROL THERAPY

The use of glycerol, a hyperosmolar agent and an osmotic diuretic, was proposed more than 30 years ago for preventing sequelae from Hib meningitis.[139] An increase in serum osmolarity has been proposed as a possible mechanism for the beneficial effect of glycerol therapy.[140] Recently, given the lack of consistent results with dexamethasone, new attention has been directed to this therapeutic strategy. In one study, oral glycerol therapy was shown to prevent severe neurologic sequelae in children with Hib meningitis. Hearing loss was, however, only slightly decreased by glycerol therapy.[137] Glycerol may represent a safe and low cost adjunct therapy in resource-limited settings with incomplete vaccination programs against Hib.[128] However, to date, there is insufficient clinical or experimental evidence to support glycerol therapy for BM.[141,142]

PERSPECTIVES AND SUMMARY

The concept that the host-mediated inflammatory reaction, in concert with bacterial factors, is responsible for the development of neurologic sequelae in BM is supported by experimental and clinical evidence. However, the appropriate strategy to circumvent these adverse events in neonatal meningitis remains to be found. Encouraging results were found in disease models evaluating the impact of pharmacologic interventions on histomorphology and neurofunctional outcomes (see **Table 1**). Changes in antibiotic choice and timing have been suggested to prevent the rapid release of proinflammatory bacterial components. In that view, the use of nonlytic antibiotics such as daptomycin or rifampin, has been shown to decrease inflammation and improve neurologic outcome. However, for empiric therapy, these "softly-killing" antibiotics need to be combined with more powerful broad-spectrum antibiotics. Sequential therapy with a nonlytic antibiotic followed by ceftriaxone yielded promising results in preliminary studies and merits further clinical evaluation. Using roscovitine to decrease the lifespan of the PMN and prevent prolonged intrathecal production of inflammatory mediators also represents a promising new avenue for therapy. More studies are needed to evaluate dosage and long-term effects.

BM is a medical emergency requiring an immediate response. A delay in the clearance of bacteria from the CSF has been shown to worsen the clinical outcome; therefore, antibiotic therapy must be started immediately.[89] Once bacteria are cleared, dynamic processes of regeneration occur in the CNS. For example, neurogenesis in the hippocampus has been shown to be increased after BM in experimental models.[143] At the transcriptomic level, dynamic changes involving the modulation of inflammatory reaction have been found during the acute phase of the disease; whereas regenerative mechanisms were initiated shortly after bacterial clearance and the resolution of the inflammation.[144,145] In addition to interventional measures during the acute phase of the disease, the development of therapies aimed at supporting neuronal repair mechanisms may hold promise to improve the long-term outcome of neonates and children with BM in the future.

REFERENCES

1. van de Beek D, de Gans J, Tunkel AR, et al. Community-acquired bacterial meningitis in adults. N Engl J Med 2006;354(1):44–53.
2. Roos KL, Van de Beek D. Bacterial meningitis. In: Roos KL, Tunkel AR, editors. Bacterial infections of the central nervous system. Amsterdam: Elsevier; 2010. p. 51–63.

3. Weisfelt M, de Gans J, van der Poll T, et al. Pneumococcal meningitis in adults: new approaches to management and prevention. Lancet Neurol 2006;5(4): 332–42.

4. Stephens DS. Conquering the meningococcus. FEMS Microbiol Rev 2007;31(1): 3–14.

5. Peltola H. Worldwide *Haemophilus influenzae* type b disease at the beginning of the 21st century: global analysis of the disease burden 25 years after the use of the polysaccharide vaccine and a decade after the advent of conjugates. Clin Microbiol Rev 2000;13(2):302–17.

6. Brouwer MC, van de Beek D, Heckenberg SG, et al. Community-acquired *Listeria monocytogenes* meningitis in adults. Clin Infect Dis 2006;43(10):1233–8.

7. Whitney CG, Farley MM, Hadler J, et al. Decline in invasive pneumococcal disease after the introduction of protein-polysaccharide conjugate vaccine. N Engl J Med 2003;348(18):1737–46.

8. Dagan R. Serotype replacement in perspective. Vaccine 2009;27(Suppl 3): C22–4.

9. Watt JP, Wolfson LJ, O'Brien KL, et al. Burden of disease caused by *Haemophilus influenzae* type b in children younger than 5 years: global estimates. Lancet 2009;374(9693):903–11.

10. O'Brien KL, Wolfson LJ, Watt JP, et al. Burden of disease caused by *Streptococcus pneumoniae* in children younger than 5 years: global estimates. Lancet 2009;374(9693):893–902.

11. Harvey D, Holt DE, Bedford H. Bacterial meningitis in the newborn: a prospective study of mortality and morbidity. Semin Perinatol 1999;23(3):218–25.

12. Bedford H, de Louvois J, Halket S, et al. Meningitis in infancy in England and Wales: follow up at age 5 years. BMJ 2001;323(7312):533–6.

13. de Louvois J, Halket S, Harvey D. Neonatal meningitis in England and Wales: sequelae at 5 years of age. Eur J Pediatr 2005;164(12):730–4.

14. Grimwood K, Anderson P, Anderson V, et al. Twelve year outcomes following bacterial meningitis: further evidence for persisting effects. Arch Dis Child 2000;83(2):111–6.

15. Anderson V, Anderson P, Grimwood K, et al. Cognitive and executive function 12 years after childhood bacterial meningitis: effect of acute neurologic complications and age of onset. J Pediatr Psychol 2004;29(2):67–81.

16. Kim YS, Sheldon RA, Elliot BR, et al. Brain damage in neonatal meningitis caused by group B streptococci in rats. J Neuropathol Exp Neurol 1995;54: 531–9.

17. Leib SL, Kim YS, Chow LL, et al. Reactive oxygen intermediates contribute to necrotic and apoptotic neuronal injury in an infant rat model of bacterial meningitis due to group B streptococci. J Clin Invest 1996;98(11):2632–9.

18. Grandgirard D, Steiner O, Täuber MG, et al. An infant mouse model of brain damage in pneumococcal meningitis. Acta Neuropathol 2007;114(6):609–17.

19. Park WS, Chang YS, Lee M. Effect of induced hyperglycemia on brain cell membrane function and energy metabolism during the early phase of experimental meningitis in newborn piglets. Brain Res 1998;798(1–2):195–203.

20. Rodriguez AF, Kaplan SL, Hawkins EP, et al. *Hematogenous pneumococcal meningitis* in the infant rat: description of a model. J Infect Dis 1991;164(6): 1207–9.

21. Kim KS, Wass CA, Cross AS. Blood-brain barrier permeability during the development of experimental bacterial meningitis in the rat. Exp Neurol 1997;145(1): 253–7.

22. Zwijnenburg PJ, van der Poll T, Florquin S, et al. Experimental pneumococcal meningitis in mice: a model of intranasal infection. J Infect Dis 2001;183(7):1143–6.
23. Leib SL, Kim YS, Ferriero DM, et al. Neuroprotective effect of excitatory amino acid antagonist kynurenic acid in experimental bacterial meningitis. J Infect Dis 1996;173(1):166–71.
24. Leib SL, Kim YS, Black SM, et al. Inducible nitric oxide synthase and the effect of aminoguanidine in experimental neonatal meningitis. J Infect Dis 1998;177(3): 692–700.
25. Michelet C, Leib SL, Bentue-Ferrer D, et al. Comparative efficacies of antibiotics in a rat model of meningoencephalitis due to *Listeria monocytogenes*. Antimicrob Agents Chemother 1999;43(7):1651–6.
26. Remer KA, Jungi TW, Fatzer R, et al. Nitric oxide is protective in listeric meningoencephalitis of rats. Infect Immun 2001;69(6):4086–93.
27. Trampuz A, Steinhuber A, Wittwer M, et al. Rapid diagnosis of experimental meningitis by bacterial heat production in cerebrospinal fluid. BMC Infect Dis 2007;7:116.
28. Leib SL, Kim YS, Black SM, et al. Detrimental effect of nitric oxide inhibition in experimental bacterial meningitis. Ann Neurol 1996;39(4):555–6.
29. Grandgirard D, Oberson K, Bühlmann A, et al. Attenuation of cerebrospinal fluid inflammation by the nonbacteriolytic antibiotic daptomycin versus that by ceftriaxone in experimental pneumococcal meningitis. Antimicrob Agents Chemother 2010;54(3):1323–6.
30. Moxon ER, Smith AL, Averill DR, et al. *Haemophilus influenzae* meningitis in infant rats after intranasal inoculation. J Infect Dis 1974;129(2):154–62.
31. Nelson E, Blinzinger K, Hager H. Ultrastructural observations on phagocytosis of bacteria in experimental (*E. coli*) meningitis. J Neuropathol Exp Neurol 1962;21:155–69.
32. Colicchio R, Ricci S, Lamberti F, et al. The meningococcal ABC-Type L-glutamate transporter GltT is necessary for the development of experimental meningitis in mice. Infect Immun 2009;77(9):3578–87.
33. Toropainen M, Kayhty H, Saarinen L, et al. The infant rat model adapted to evaluate human sera for protective immunity to group B meningococci. Vaccine 1999;17(20–21):2677–89.
34. Salit IE, Tomalty L. A neonatal mouse model of meningococcal disease. Clin Invest Med 1986;9(2):119–23.
35. Hill DJ, Griffiths NJ, Borodina E, et al. Cellular and molecular biology of *Neisseria meningitidis* colonization and invasive disease. Clin Sci (Lond) 2010;118(9): 547–64.
36. Bevanger L, Bergh K, Gisnas G, et al. Identification of nasopharyngeal carriage of an outbreak strain of *Neisseria meningitidis* by pulsed-field gel electrophoresis versus phenotypic methods. J Med Microbiol 1998;47(11):993–8.
37. Tzeng YL, Stephens DS. Epidemiology and pathogenesis of *Neisseria meningitidis*. Microbes Infect 2000;2(6):687–700.
38. Schwartz B. Chemoprophylaxis for bacterial infections: principles of and application to meningococcal infections. Rev Infect Dis 1991;13(Suppl 2):S170–3.
39. Garcia-Rodriguez JA, Fresnadillo Martinez MJ. Dynamics of nasopharyngeal colonization by potential respiratory pathogens. J Antimicrob Chemother 2002;50(Suppl S2):59–73.
40. Leib SL, Täuber MG. Pathogenesis and pathophysiology of bacterial infections. In: Scheld WM, Whitley RJ, Marra CM, editors. Infections of the central nervous system. 3rd edition. Philadelphia: Lippincott Williams & Wilkins; 2004. p. 331–46.

41. Kim KS. Acute bacterial meningitis in infants and children. Lancet Infect Dis 2010;10(1):32–42.
42. Kim KS. Mechanisms of microbial traversal of the blood-brain barrier. Nat Rev Microbiol 2008;6(8):625–34.
43. Antal EA, Loberg EM, Bracht P, et al. Evidence for intraaxonal spread of *Listeria monocytogenes* from the periphery to the central nervous system. Brain Pathol 2001;11(4):432–8.
44. Kastenbauer S, Pfister HW. Pneumococcal meningitis in adults: spectrum of complications and prognostic factors in a series of 87 cases. Brain 2003; 126(Pt 5):1015–25.
45. Small PM, Täuber MG, Hackbarth CJ, et al. Influence of body temperature on bacterial growth rates in experimental pneumococcal meningitis in rabbits. Infect Immun 1986;52:484–7.
46. Koedel U, Klein M, Pfister HW. New understandings on the pathophysiology of bacterial meningitis. Curr Opin Infect Dis 2010;23(3):217–23.
47. Koedel U. Toll-like receptors in bacterial meningitis. Curr Top Microbiol Immunol 2009;336:15–40.
48. Opitz B, Puschel A, Schmeck B, et al. Nucleotide-binding oligomerization domain proteins are innate immune receptors for internalized *Streptococcus pneumoniae*. J Biol Chem 2004;279(35):36426–32.
49. Sellner J, Täuber MG, Leib SL. Pathogenesis and pathophysiology of bacterial CNS infection. In: Roos KL, Tunkel AR, editors. Bacterial infections of the central nervous system. Amsterdam: Elsevier; 2010. p. 1–16.
50. Zwijnenburg PJ, van der Poll T, Roord JJ, et al. Chemotactic factors in cerebrospinal fluid during bacterial meningitis. Infect Immun 2006;74(3):1445–51.
51. Ostergaard C, Benfield TL, Sellebjerg F, et al. Interleukin-8 in cerebrospinal fluid from patients with septic and aseptic meningitis. Eur J Clin Microbiol Infect Dis 1996;15(2):166–9.
52. Zwijnenburg PJ, de Bie HM, Roord JJ, et al. Chemotactic activity of CXCL5 in cerebrospinal fluid of children with bacterial meningitis. J Neuroimmunol 2003; 145(1–2):148–53.
53. Sellner J, Leib SL. In bacterial meningitis cortical brain damage is associated with changes in parenchymal MMP-9/TIMP-1 ratio and increased collagen type IV degradation. Neurobiol Dis 2006;21(3):647–56.
54. Leppert D, Leib SL, Grygar C, et al. Matrix metalloproteinase (MMP)-8 and MMP-9 in cerebrospinal fluid during bacterial meningitis: association with blood-brain barrier damage and neurological sequelae. Clin Infect Dis 2000;31(1):80–4.
55. Kastenbauer S, Koedel U, Becker BF, et al. Oxidative stress in bacterial meningitis in humans. Neurology 2002;58(2):186–91.
56. Schaper M, Gergely S, Lykkesfeldt J, et al. Cerebral vasculature is the major target of oxidative protein alterations in bacterial meningitis. J Neuropathol Exp Neurol 2002;61(7):605–13.
57. Ghielmetti M, Ren H, Leib SL, et al. Impaired cortical energy metabolism but not major antioxidant defenses in experimental bacterial meningitis. Brain Res 2003; 976(2):139–48.
58. Koedel U, Winkler F, Angele B, et al. Meningitis-associated central nervous system complications are mediated by the activation of poly(ADP-ribose) polymerase. J Cereb Blood Flow Metab 2002;22(1):39–49.
59. Anderson V, Bond L, Catroppa C, et al. Childhood bacterial meningitis: impact of age at illness and acute medical complications on long term outcome. J Int Neuropsychol Soc 1997;3(2):147–58.

60. Weisfelt M, van de Beek D, Spanjaard L, et al. Clinical features, complications, and outcome in adults with pneumococcal meningitis: a prospective case series. Lancet Neurol 2006;5(2):123–9.
61. Takeoka M, Takahashi T. Infectious and inflammatory disorders of the circulatory system and stroke in childhood. Curr Opin Neurol 2002;15(2):159–64.
62. Pfister LA, Tureen JH, Shaw S, et al. Endothelin inhibition improves cerebral blood flow and is neuroprotective in pneumococcal meningitis. Ann Neurol 2000;47(3):329–35.
63. Koedel U, Scheld WM, Pfister HW. Pathogenesis and pathophysiology of pneumococcal meningitis. Lancet Infect Dis 2002;2(12):721–36.
64. Berman PH, Banker BQ. Neonatal meningitis. A clinical and pathological study of 29 cases. Pediatrics 1966;38:6–24.
65. Grandgirard D, Schurch C, Cottagnoud P, et al. Prevention of brain injury by the nonbacteriolytic antibiotic daptomycin in experimental pneumococcal meningitis. Antimicrob Agents Chemother 2007;51(6):2173–8.
66. Leib SL, Clements JM, Lindberg RL, et al. Inhibition of matrix metalloproteinases and tumour necrosis factor alpha converting enzyme as adjuvant therapy in pneumococcal meningitis. Brain 2001;124(Pt 9):1734–42.
67. Leib SL, Heimgartner C, Bifrare YD, et al. Dexamethasone aggravates hippocampal apoptosis and learning deficiency in pneumococcal meningitis in infant rats. Pediatr Res 2003;4:4.
68. Loeffler JM, Ringer R, Hablutzel M, et al. The free radical scavenger alpha-phenyl-tert-butyl nitrone aggravates hippocampal apoptosis and learning deficits in experimental pneumococcal meningitis. J Infect Dis 2001;183(2):247–52.
69. Wellmer A, Noeske C, Gerber J, et al. Spatial memory and learning deficits after experimental pneumococcal meningitis in mice. Neurosci Lett 2000;296(2–3):137–40.
70. Gianinazzi C, Grandgirard D, Imboden H, et al. Caspase-3 mediates hippocampal apoptosis in pneumococcal meningitis. Acta Neuropathol 2003;105:499–507.
71. Nau R, Soto A, Bruck W. Apoptosis of neurons in the dentate gyrus in humans suffering from bacterial meningitis. J Neuropathol Exp Neurol 1999;58(3):265–74.
72. Grandgirard D, Bifrare YD, Pleasure SJ, et al. Pneumococcal meningitis induces apoptosis in recently postmitotic immature neurons in the dentate gyrus of neonatal rats. Dev Neurosci 2007;29(1–2):134–42.
73. Sury MD, Agarinis C, Widmer HR, et al. JNK is activated but does not mediate hippocampal neuronal apoptosis in experimental neonatal pneumococcal meningitis. Neurobiol Dis 2008;32(1):142–50.
74. Hofer S, Grandgirard D, Trachsel T, et al. Apoptosis of neurogenic cells in an in vitro model of bacterial meningitis. 20th European Congress of Clinical Microbiology and Infectious Diseases (ECCMID). Vienna (Austria), April 10–13, 2010.
75. Bifrare YD, Gianinazzi C, Imboden H, et al. Bacterial meningitis causes two distinct forms of cellular damage in the hippocampal dentate gyrus in infant rats. Hippocampus 2003;13(4):481–8.
76. van der Flier M, Geelen SP, Kimpen JL, et al. Reprogramming the host response in bacterial meningitis: how best to improve outcome? Clin Microbiol Rev 2003;16(3):415–29.
77. Meli DN, Christen S, Leib SL, et al. Current concepts in the pathogenesis of meningitis caused by *Streptococcus pneumoniae*. Curr Opin Infect Dis 2002;15(3):253–7.

78. Ostergaard C, Leib SL, Rowland I, et al. Bacteremia causes hippocampal apoptosis in experimental pneumococcal meningitis. BMC Infect Dis 2010; 10:1.
79. Semmler A, Okulla T, Sastre M, et al. Systemic inflammation induces apoptosis with variable vulnerability of different brain regions. J Chem Neuroanat 2005; 30(2–3):144–57.
80. Yagita Y, Kitagawa K, Ohtsuki T, et al. Neurogenesis by progenitor cells in the ischemic adult rat hippocampus. Stroke 2001;32(8):1890–6.
81. Cameron HA, Woolley CS, McEwen BS, et al. Differentiation of newly born neurons and glia in the dentate gyrus of the adult rat. Neuroscience 1993; 56(2):337–44.
82. Eriksson PS, Perfilieva E, Bjork-Eriksson T, et al. Neurogenesis in the adult human hippocampus. Nat Med 1998;4(11):1313–7.
83. de Jonge RC, Swart JF, Koomen I, et al. No structural cerebral differences between children with a history of bacterial meningitis and healthy siblings. Acta Paediatr 2008;97(10):1390–6.
84. van de Beek D, de Gans J. Meningitis-associated hearing loss: protection by adjunctive antioxidant therapy. Ann Neurol 2004;55(4):597–8 [author reply 8].
85. Kaplan SL, Catlin FI, Weaver T, et al. Onset of hearing loss in children with bacterial meningitis. Pediatrics 1984;73(5):575–8.
86. Klein M, Koedel U, Kastenbauer S, et al. Nitrogen and oxygen molecules in meningitis-associated labyrinthitis and hearing impairment. Infection 2008; 36(1):2–14.
87. Klein M, Koedel U, Pfister H-W, et al. Morphological correlates of acute and permanent hearing loss during experimental pneumococcal meningitis. Brain Pathol 2003;13:123–32.
88. Grandgirard D, Leib SL. Strategies to prevent neuronal damage in paediatric bacterial meningitis. Curr Opin Pediatr 2006;18(2):112–8.
89. Klein M, Pfister HW, Leib SL, et al. Therapy of community-acquired acute bacterial meningitis: the clock is running. Expert Opin Pharmacother 2009;10(16): 2609–23.
90. Mustafa MM, Mertsola J, Ramilo O, et al. Increased endotoxin and interleukin-1 beta concentrations in cerebrospinal fluid of infants with coliform meningitis and ventriculitis associated with intraventricular gentamicin therapy. J Infect Dis 1989;160(5):891–5.
91. Täuber MG, Shibl AM, Hackbarth CJ, et al. Antibiotic therapy, endotoxin concentration in cerebrospinal fluid, and brain edema in experimental *Escherichia coli* meningitis in rabbits. J Infect Dis 1987;156(3):456–62.
92. Nau R, Eiffert H. Minimizing the release of proinflammatory and toxic bacterial products within the host: a promising approach to improve outcome in life-threatening infections. FEMS Immunol Med Microbiol 2005;44(1):1–16.
93. Gerber J, Pohl K, Sander V, et al. Rifampin followed by ceftriaxone for experimental meningitis decreases lipoteichoic acid concentrations in cerebrospinal fluid and reduces neuronal damage in comparison to ceftriaxone alone. Antimicrob Agents Chemother 2003;47(4):1313–7.
94. Spreer A, Lugert R, Stoltefaut V, et al. Short-term rifampicin pretreatment reduces inflammation and neuronal cell death in a rabbit model of bacterial meningitis. Crit Care Med 2009;37(7):2253–8.
95. Bottcher T, Ren H, Goiny M, et al. Clindamycin is neuroprotective in experimental *Streptococcus pneumoniae* meningitis compared with ceftriaxone. J Neurochem 2004;91(6):1450–60.

96. Stucki A, Cottagnoud M, Winkelmann V, et al. Daptomycin produces an enhanced bactericidal activity compared to ceftriaxone, measured by [3H]choline release in the cerebrospinal fluid, in experimental meningitis due to a penicillin-resistant pneumococcal strain without lysing its cell wall. Antimicrob Agents Chemother 2007;51(6):2249–52.

97. Egermann U, Stanga Z, Ramin A, et al. The combination of daptomycin plus ceftriaxone was more active than vancomycin plus ceftriaxone in experimental meningitis after addition of dexamethasone. Antimicrob Agents Chemother 2009;53(7):3030–3.

98. Grandgirard D, Burri D, Oberson K, et al. In infant rat pneumococcal meningitis, ceftriaxone plus daptomycin versus ceftriaxone attenuates brain damage and hearing loss while ceftriaxone plus rifampicin versus ceftriaxone does not. 19th European Congress of Clinical Microbiology and Infectious Diseases (ECCMID). Helsinki (Finnland), May 16–19, 2009.

99. Meli DN, Loeffler JM, Baumann P, et al. In pneumococcal meningitis a novel water-soluble inhibitor of matrix metalloproteinases and TNF-alpha converting enzyme attenuates seizures and injury of the cerebral cortex. J Neuroimmunol 2004;151(1–2):6–11.

100. Meli DN, Coimbra RS, Erhart DG, et al. Doxycycline reduces mortality and injury to the brain and cochlea in experimental pneumococcal meningitis. Infect Immun 2006;74(7):3890–6.

101. Auer M, Pfister LA, Leppert D, et al. Effects of clinically used antioxidants in experimental pneumococcal meningitis. J Infect Dis 2000;182(1):347–50.

102. Klein M, Koedel U, Pfister HW, et al. Meningitis-associated hearing loss: protection by adjunctive antioxidant therapy. Ann Neurol 2003;54(4):451–8.

103. Ge NN, Brodie HA, Tinling SP. Long-term hearing loss in gerbils with bacterial meningitis treated with superoxide dismutase. Otol Neurotol 2008;31(3):394–403.

104. Spreer A, Gerber J, Baake D, et al. Antiinflammatory but no neuroprotective effects of melatonin under clinical treatment conditions in rabbit models of bacterial meningitis. J Neurosci Res 2006;84(7):1575–9.

105. Ostergaard C, Yieng-Kow RV, Benfield T, et al. Inhibition of leukocyte entry into the brain by the selectin blocker fucoidin decreases interleukin-1 (IL-1) levels but increases IL-8 levels in cerebrospinal fluid during experimental pneumococcal meningitis in rabbits. Infect Immun 2000;68(6):3153–7.

106. Brandt CT, Lundgren JD, Frimodt-Moller N, et al. Blocking of leukocyte accumulation in the cerebrospinal fluid augments bacteremia and increases lethality in experimental pneumococcal meningitis. J Neuroimmunol 2005;166(1–2):126–31.

107. Brandt CT, Lundgren JD, Lund SP, et al. Attenuation of the bacterial load in blood by pretreatment with granulocyte-colony-stimulating factor protects rats from fatal outcome and brain damage during Streptococcus pneumoniae meningitis. Infect Immun 2004;72(8):4647–53.

108. Brandt CT, Caye-Thomasen P, Lund SP, et al. Hearing loss and cochlear damage in experimental pneumococcal meningitis, with special reference to the role of neutrophil granulocytes. Neurobiol Dis 2006;23(2):300–11.

109. Koedel U, Frankenberg T, Kirschnek S, et al. Apoptosis is essential for neutrophil functional shutdown and determines tissue damage in experimental pneumococcal meningitis. PLoS Pathog 2009;5(5):e1000461.

110. Rossi AG, Sawatzky DA, Walker A, et al. Cyclin-dependent kinase inhibitors enhance the resolution of inflammation by promoting inflammatory cell apoptosis. Nat Med 2006;12(9):1056–64.

111. Thornberry NA, Lazebnik Y. Caspases: enemies within. Science 1998; 281(5381):1312–6.
112. Braun JS, Novak R, Herzog KH, et al. Neuroprotection by a caspase inhibitor in acute bacterial meningitis. Nat Med 1999;5(3):298–302.
113. Bifrare YD, Kummer J, Joss P, et al. Brain-derived neurotrophic factor protects against multiple forms of brain injury in bacterial meningitis. J Infect Dis 2005; 191(1):40–5.
114. Li L, Shui QX, Zhao ZY. Regulation of brain-derived neurotrophic factor (BDNF) expression following antibiotic treatment of experimental bacterial meningitis. J Child Neurol 2003;18(12):828–34.
115. Li L, Shui QX, Li X. Neuroprotective effects of brain-derived neurotrophic factor (BDNF) on hearing in experimental pneumococcal meningitis. J Child Neurol 2005;20(1):51–6.
116. Sola A, Wen TC, Hamrick SE, et al. Potential for protection and repair following injury to the developing brain: a role for erythropoietin? Pediatr Res 2005;57(5 Pt 2):110R–7.
117. Wen TC, Sadamoto Y, Tanaka J, et al. Erythropoietin protects neurons against chemical hypoxia and cerebral ischemic injury by up-regulating Bcl-xL expression. J Neurosci Res 2002;67(6):795–803.
118. Spreer A, Gerber J, Hanssen M, et al. No neuroprotective effect of erythropoietin under clinical treatment conditions in a rabbit model of *Escherichia coli* meningitis. Pediatr Res 2007;62(6):680–3.
119. Kastenbauer S, Koedel U, Becker BF, et al. Pneumococcal meningitis in the rat: evaluation of peroxynitrite scavengers for adjunctive therapy. Eur J Pharmacol 2002;449(1–2):177–81.
120. Kastenbauer S, Koedel U, Becker BF, et al. Experimental meningitis in the rat: protection by uric acid at human physiological blood concentrations. Eur J Pharmacol 2001;425(2):149–52.
121. Pfister HW, Kodel U, Dirnagl U, et al. Effect of catalase on regional cerebral blood flow and brain edema during the early phase of experimental pneumococcal meningitis. J Infect Dis 1992;166(6):1442–5.
122. Kastenbauer S, Koedel U, Pfister HW. Role of peroxynitrite as a mediator of pathophysiological alterations in experimental pneumococcal meningitis. J Infect Dis 1999;180(4):1164–70.
123. Koedel U, Pfister HW. Protective effect of the antioxidant N-acetyl-L-cysteine in pneumococcal meningitis in the rat. Neurosci Lett 1997;225(1):33–6.
124. Klein M, Koedel U, Pfister HW. Oxidative stress in pneumococcal meningitis: a future target for adjunctive therapy? Prog Neurobiol 2006;80(6): 269–80.
125. Koedel U, Gorriz C, Lorenzl S, et al. Increased endothelin levels in cerebrospinal fluid samples from adults with bacterial meningitis. Clin Infect Dis 1997;25(2): 329–30.
126. Tureen JH, Täuber MG, Sande MA. Effect of indomethacin on the pathophysiology of experimental meningitis in rabbits. J Infect Dis 1991;163(3):647–9.
127. van de Beek D, Farrar JJ, de Gans J, et al. Adjunctive dexamethasone in bacterial meningitis: a meta-analysis of individual patient data. Lancet Neurol 2010; 9(3):254–63.
128. Peltola H, Roine I, Fernandez J, et al. Adjuvant glycerol and/or dexamethasone to improve the outcomes of childhood bacterial meningitis: a prospective, randomized, double-blind, placebo-controlled trial. Clin Infect Dis 2007; 45(10):1277–86.

129. Spreer A, Gerber J, Hanssen M, et al. Dexamethasone increases hippocampal neuronal apoptosis in a rabbit model of *Escherichia coli* meningitis. Pediatr Res 2006;60(2):210–5.

130. Irazuzta J, Pretzlaff RK, DeCourten-Myers G, et al. Dexamethasone decreases neurological sequelae and caspase activity. Intensive Care Med 2005;31(1): 146–50.

131. Coimbra RS, Loquet G, Leib SL. Limited efficacy of adjuvant therapy with dexamethasone in preventing hearing loss due to experimental pneumococcal meningitis in the infant rat. Pediatr Res 2007;62(3):291–4.

132. Worsoe L, Brandt CT, Lund SP, et al. Intratympanic steroid prevents long-termspiral ganglion neuron loss in experimental meningitis. Otol Neurotol 2010;31(3):394–403.

133. Addison J, Kim HH, Richter CP. Cochlear preservation after meningitis: an animal model confirmation of adjunctive steroid therapy. Laryngoscope 2006; 116(2):279–82.

134. Rappaport JM, Bhatt SM, Burkard RF, et al. Prevention of hearing loss in experimental pneumococcal meningitis by administration of dexamethasone and ketorolac. J Infect Dis 1999;179(1):264–8.

135. McIntyre PB, Berkey CS, King SM, et al. Dexamethasone as adjunctive therapy in bacterial meningitis. A meta-analysis of randomized clinical trials since 1988. JAMA 1997;278(11):925–31.

136. Molyneux EM, Walsh AL, Forsyth H, et al. Dexamethasone treatment in childhood bacterial meningitis in Malawi: a randomised controlled trial. Lancet 2002;360(9328):211–8.

137. Peltola H, Roine I, Fernandez J, et al. Hearing impairment in childhood bacterial meningitis is little relieved by dexamethasone or glycerol. Pediatrics 2010; 125(1):e1–8.

138. Assiri AM, Alasmari FA, Zimmerman VA, et al. Corticosteroid administration and outcome of adolescents and adults with acute bacterial meningitis: a meta-analysis. Mayo Clin Proc 2009;84(5):403–9.

139. Herson VC, Todd JK. Prediction of morbidity in *Hemophilus influenzae* meningitis. Pediatrics 1977;59(1):35–9.

140. Singhi S, Jarvinen A, Peltola H. Increase in serum osmolality is possible mechanism for the beneficial effects of glycerol in childhood bacterial meningitis. Pediatr Infect Dis J 2008;27(10):892–6.

141. Blaser C, Klein M, Grandgirard D, et al. Adjuvant glyerol is not beneficial in experimental pneumococcal meningitis. BMC Infect Dis 2010;10:84.

142. Schmidt H, Stuertz K, Chen V, et al. Glycerol does not reduce neuronal damage in experimental *Streptococcus pneumoniae* meningitis in rabbits 1998;6(1):19–26.

143. Täuber SC, Stadelmann C, Spreer A, et al. Increased expression of BDNF and proliferation of dentate granule cells after bacterial meningitis. J Neuropathol Exp Neurol 2005;64(9):806–15.

144. Wittwer M, Grandgirard D, Rohrbach J, Leib SL. Tracking the transcriptional host response from the acute to the regenerative phase of experimental pneumococcal meningitis. BMC Infect Dis 2010. 10:176. [Online].

145. Coimbra RS, Voisin V, de Saizieu AB, et al. Gene expression in cortex and hippocampus during acute pneumococcal meningitis. BMC Biol 2006;4(1):15.

146. Nau R, Bruck W. Neuronal injury in bacterial meningitis: mechanisms and implications for therapy. Trends Neurosci 2002;25(1):38–45.

147. Kastenbauer S, Klein M, Koedel U, et al. Reactive nitrogen species contribute to blood-labyrinth barrier disruption in suppurative labyrinthitis complicating

experimental pneumococcal meningitis in the rat. Brain Res 2001;904(2): 208–17.

148. Leib SL, Leppert D, Clements J, et al. Matrix metalloproteinases contribute to brain damage in experimental pneumococcal meningitis. Infect Immun 2000; 68(2):615–20.

149. Bogdan I, Leib SL, Bergeron M, et al. Tumor necrosis factor-alpha contributes to apoptosis in hippocampal neurons during experimental group B streptococcal meningitis. J Infect Dis 1997;176(3):693–7.

150. Sellner J, Ringer R, Baumann P, et al. Effect of the NMDA-receptor antagonist dextromethorphan in infant rat pneumococcal meningitis. Curr Drug Metab 2008;9(1):83–8.

151. Kolarova A, Ringer R, Tauber MG, et al. Blockade of NMDA receptor subtype NR2B prevents seizures but not apoptosis of dentate gyrus neurons in bacterial meningitis in infant rats. BMC Neurosci 2003;4(1):21.

Progress Toward Improved Understanding of Infection-Related Preterm Birth

Tara M. Randis, MD

KEYWORDS

- Preterm birth • Chorioamnionitis • Bacterial vaginosis
- Fetal inflammatory response

The association between chorioamnionitis and preterm labor has long been recognized.[1,2] However, existing strategies to prevent infection-related preterm birth and the associated neonatal morbidities have met with limited success.[3–6] Potential reasons for this include (1) failure to diagnose occult intra-amniotic infections, (2) starting therapy long after injurious inflammatory processes are underway, (3) low bioavailability of antibiotics in amniotic fluid and/or fetal tissues, and (4) additional host factors, such as diet, smoking, and genetic variations in inflammatory response.[7–9] Acute chorioamnionitis is a response to microbial invasion of the amniotic fluid,[10] generally by organisms known to colonize the lower genital tract. The microorganisms most commonly associated with preterm birth and chorioamnionitis are genital *Mycoplasma* sp, *Ureaplasma* sp, *Mobiluncus* sp, *Bacteroides* sp, group B β-hemolytic streptococci, and *Gardnerella vaginalis*.[11–13] A recent review by Iams and colleagues[14] suggests that the association between preterm birth and microorganisms colonizing and infecting the genital tract must be further elucidated before antimicrobial agents can be used effectively and safely to prevent preterm birth.

Over the last decade, notable progress has been made in our understanding of altered genital tract colonization, namely bacterial vaginosis (BV), and how this may contribute to the onset of preterm labor. The application of novel molecular techniques to diagnose intra-amniotic infection allows for a greater appreciation of the absolute magnitude of the problem and improved identification of those women who may benefit most from antimicrobial therapy. Increased recognition of the fetal inflammatory

The author has nothing to disclose.
Division of Neonatology, Columbia University Medical Center, 3959 Broadway, CHN 1201, New York, NY 10032, USA
E-mail address: tmr2103@columbia.edu

Clin Perinatol 37 (2010) 677–688
doi:10.1016/j.clp.2010.06.001
0095-5108/10/$ – see front matter © 2010 Elsevier Inc. All rights reserved.

response to intrauterine pathogens has clarified the pathophysiologic mechanisms underlying infection-related preterm birth and postnatal consequences, including potentially altered susceptibility to common neonatal pathogens.

BV: RECENT DEVELOPMENTS

BV is a pathologic state characterized by the loss of normal vaginal flora, particularly *Lactobacillus* species, and overgrowth of other microbes, including *G vaginalis, Bacteroides* sp, *Mobiluncus* sp, and *Mycoplasma hominis*. Reported prevalence rates for BV range from 10% to 40% depending on the population studied, with the vast majority of women being asymptomatic.[15,16] BV during pregnancy is an independent risk factor for preterm labor[17] and is estimated to cause 90,000 excess premature births per year and to account for at least 30% of the racial difference in preterm birth rates.[15] Although BV in pregnant women can be successfully treated using appropriate antimicrobial therapy, several large clinical trials have demonstrated that the use of antibiotics in these women has not been associated with reduced preterm births.[18,19] Until understanding of the bacterial-host interaction improves, further interventions directed at reducing BV-associated preterm births are unlikely to succeed.[20]

The mechanism by which BV leads to preterm birth has not yet been elucidated. It is likely secondary to ascent of vaginal microorganisms into the uterus before or early during pregnancy since, BV-associated bacteria are recovered from the amniotic fluid and chorioamnion of patients who deliver prematurely.[20–22] It is hypothesized that the host inflammatory response to these organisms stimulates the release of inflammatory mediators, such as interleukin (IL)-1β and IL-8, that contribute to the onset of preterm labor.[23–25] The inflammation associated with BV may not be limited to maternal tissues, as there is now evidence to suggest that alterations in vaginal microbiota influence the fetal cytokine profile in cord blood.[26]

BV is best understood as a polymicrobial disease; however, recent data suggest a critical role for *G vaginalis* as the primary, sexually transmitted agent, which was initially postulated by Gardner and Dukes in 1955.[27–29] Gelber and colleagues[30] recently identified and characterized vaginolysin (VLY), a novel pore-forming toxin produced by *G vaginalis,* which is hypothesized to be a major factor in the pathogenesis of BV and its associated morbidities. VLY is capable of eliciting proinflammatory signaling in host epithelial cells, including phosphorylation of p38 mitogen-activated protein kinase, processing and subsequent upregulation of pro-IL-1β, and induction of IL-8 transcripts.[30] The pore-forming activity of this toxin is human-specific, using the glycosylphosphatidyl-inositol–anchored protein CD59 as its receptor. This requirement for human CD59 may explain the lack of a suitable animal model of BV. The functional characterization of VLY represents an important step in our understanding of the critical bacterial-host interactions in the pathogenesis of BV. Furthermore, antibody-based strategies have been successfully used for detection and quantification of VLY production in vivo and inhibition of its toxic effects on human cells. These strategies may have a potential role in the diagnosis and treatment of BV.

Black race, low educational attainment, increasing number of sexual partners, and douching have all been associated with an increased risk for BV in nonpregnant women.[16,31] Exploration of predisposing factors in pregnant women has yielded variable results.[32–34] Recently, Bodnar and colleagues[35] indentified vitamin D deficiency as a risk factor for the development of BV in pregnant women. It is now well recognized that vitamin D is an important regulator of host immune responses, and vitamin D deficiency has been associated with increased susceptibility to numerous other infectious diseases.[36–38] Binding of 1, 25-dihydroxyvitamin D, the hormonally active vitamin D metabolite, to its nuclear receptor ultimately results in the transcription of hundreds of target genes, many of which are integral components of the innate immune system.[39] Therefore, vitamin D may locally regulate host immune signaling.[40] Altered immunity in the vaginal microenvironment provides a potential mechanistic explanation for the observed association between vitamin D deficiency and the development of BV.

These findings have enormous implications in light of the overall prevalence of vitamin D deficiency in the United States, estimated to be a staggering 77%.[41] Furthermore, serum vitamin D levels are lowest in non-Hispanic black women aged 12 to 59 years, a critical finding that may explain the profound racial disparities observed in epidemiologic studies of BV and BV-associated preterm birth.[41] The identification of potentially modifiable risk factors for BV represents a unique opportunity to reduce the burden of this exceedingly prevalent disease and its associated morbidities.

IMPROVED IDENTIFICATION OF INTRAUTERINE INFECTION

Intrauterine infection is believed to account for 25% to 40% of preterm births.[42] However, the true prevalence of infection-associated preterm labor is likely to be grossly underestimated since these approximations rely primarily on traditional diagnostic strategies, including culture-based techniques, clinical criteria, or laboratory analysis of amniotic fluid. Standard culture-based techniques often do not identify fastidious organisms or other cultivation-resistant microbes. Also, many of the organisms typically associated with the onset of preterm labor may produce clinically silent infection.

Advancements in molecular biology, such as broad-range PCR, have resulted in increased recognition of occult intrauterine infections. Broad-range PCR uses primers that recognize highly conserved sequences in bacterial species, such as those encoding for ribosomal DNA, while simultaneously amplifying highly variable regions located between the primer binding sites. The amplification product is sequenced and then compared with existing genomic libraries to identify known pathogens and previously uncharacterized bacteria.[43,44]

DiGiulio and colleagues[45] used a broad-range PCR method[46,47] to investigate microbial prevalence and diversity in the amniotic fluid of women in spontaneous preterm labor with intact membranes. These investigators demonstrated that the microbial prevalence in the amniotic fluid as determined by broad-range PCR was 56% higher than that found by routine cultivation methods. Also, PCR analysis revealed greater microbial diversity in the positive specimens than did culture alone, including several unusual organisms and one previously uncharacterized bacterial species. These investigators went on to highlight the clinical relevance of their findings by demonstrating that a positive PCR result was associated with histologic chorioamnionitis/funisitis and had a 100% positive predictive value for preterm delivery in this cohort (**Table 1**).

Han and colleagues[48] similarly analyzed the amniotic fluid of women presenting with preterm labor for the presence of bacteria not identifiable by standard culture techniques. They reported that nearly two-thirds of the species detected by PCR techniques were not identified using culture alone. Similar to DiGiulio and colleagues, these investigators were able to demonstrate that PCR analysis revealed greater microbial diversity than did culture alone. Furthermore, the presence of bacterial DNA was associated with the presence of proteomic biomarkers characteristic of intrauterine inflammation, highlighting the clinical relevance of these uncultivated species. These investigators found no bacterial DNA in the amniotic fluid of

Table 1
PPV of amniotic fluid PCR and culture for pregnancy outcomes

Outcome	Preterm Delivery (<37 weeks)	Very Preterm Delivery (<32 Weeks)	Extremely Preterm Delivery (<25 Weeks)	Delivery within One Day of Amniocentesis
Prevalence	68% (113/166)	49% (58/118)	40% (17/43)	17% (28/166)
PPV of PCR	100% (19/19)	100% (16/16)	100% (8/8)	68% (13/19)
PPV of culture	100% (16/16)	100% (14/14)	89% (8/9)	69% (11/16)
PPV of PCR and culture combined	100% (10/10)	100% (8/8)	100% (5/5)	100% (10/10)

Abbreviation: PPV, positive predictive value.
From DiGiulio DB, Romero R, Amogan HP, et al. Microbial prevalence, diversity and abundance in amniotic fluid during preterm labor: a molecular and culture-based investigation. PLoS One 2008;3:e3056; with permission.

asymptomatic controls. The use of broad-range PCR to identify bacterial DNA in the amniotic fluid has increased our understanding of the diversity and abundance of microbial species invading the amniotic cavity in the setting of preterm labor, and it may allow for more timely intervention and appropriate antibiotic selection.

Current evidence suggests that much of the morbidity observed in preterm infants is secondary to the inflammatory response to infection rather than simply being the result of premature, underdeveloped organ systems.[49,50] Accurate identification of intrauterine inflammation rather than bacterial infection may be more important in the search to develop targeted treatments.[51] The inflammatory response following microbial invasion of the amniotic cavity is characterized by the release of cytokines, recruitment of immune cells, and subsequent release of antimicrobial peptides, resulting in an altered protein composition of the amniotic fluid, which precedes overt clinical signs and symptoms.[52,53] Proteomic analysis of the amniotic fluid may thus be of benefit in early diagnosis of intrauterine infection. Furthermore, a proteomics-based approach will identify intrauterine inflammatory response in women with microbial infection as well those women with inflammation secondary to other noninfectious processes.[53]

Using surface-enhanced laser desorption/ionization time of flight, a proteomics technology that combines chromatography with mass spectrometry,[54] Buhimschi and colleagues[51] demonstrated that patients with intra-amniotic inflammation who deliver preterm have a distinctive amniotic fluid proteomic profile consisting of 3 or 4 of the following proteins: neutrophil defensin-1 and -2 and calgranulins A and C. The investigators developed the mass-restricted (MR) score based on the presence or absence of these biomarkers. They subsequently demonstrated that this scoring system was effective in identifying intra-amniotic inflammation in women with preterm labor and was predictive of imminent preterm delivery.[55] Subsequent studies by these investigators have demonstrated that when compared with other laboratory tests routinely used to diagnose amniotic fluid inflammation and infection (amniotic fluid glucose, WBC, LDH, IL-6 and matrix metalloprotease-8), the MR score had the highest accuracy in detecting inflammation, whereas the combination of Gram stain and MR score was best for rapid prediction of intra-amniotic infection.[56] Furthermore, neonates born to women with abnormal MR scores had an increased incidence of funisitis and early-onset sepsis, even after adjusting for gestational age at birth.[55,56]

Although the data from these proteomic studies are promising, the required instruments and technical skills currently preclude the adoption of these methodologies in clinical practice. However, biomarkers identified through these analyses may serve as the basis for the development of rapid cost-effective immunoassays for the diagnosis of intrauterine infections.[57] Use of proteomic profiling techniques to analyze cervicovaginal secretions rather than amniotic fluid may serve as a noninvasive alternative for diagnosing intrauterine inflammation.[58–60]

THE FETAL RESPONSE TO MATERNAL INFECTION

The fetus is capable of mounting an immune response following perturbations in the intrauterine environment. Elevated plasma concentrations of IL-6 and C-reactive protein (CRP) and a higher percentage of Th1 cells have all been documented in fetuses with preterm labor and preterm premature rupture of membranes (PROM).[61–64] However, it was not until 1998 that Gomez and colleagues[64] formally described the fetal inflammatory response syndrome (FIRS) as a condition characterized by systemic activation of the fetal immune system and defined by elevated IL-6 concentrations in neonatal cord blood.[64] These investigators determined that a cord blood IL-6 concentration of 11 pg/mL or greater was associated with microbial invasion of the amniotic cavity as documented by positive amniotic fluid culture. In their cohort of 157 women with preterm labor or preterm PROM, elevated IL-6 was an independent predictor of later neonatal morbidity.

The presence of funisitis and chorionic vasculitis are generally considered the histologic manifestations of FIRS,[65] though the pattern is somewhat dependent on gestational age. Fetal inflammatory responses in preterm placentas first appear in the chorionic plate, whereas those in term placentas are often first observed in the umbilical vein.[66] In both cases, involvement of the umbilical artery follows as inflammation progresses.[66] Fetal inflammatory responses (as opposed to maternal inflammatory responses) are rarely seen in placentas with histologic chorioamnionitis at less than 20 weeks' gestation.[66]

To identify the key biologic processes involved in FIRS, Madsen-Bouterse and colleagues[67] examined genome-wide expression in preterm neonates with evidence of inflammation in utero (defined by the presence of funisitis and elevated cord blood IL-6 concentrations). Microarray analysis was used to examine fetal leukocyte RNA obtained from umbilical vein cord blood of these neonates at the time of delivery. Critical genes involved in antigen processing and leukocyte adhesion and chemotaxis and those encoding for antimicrobial peptides were all upregulated in the setting of FIRS. The investigators concluded that the differential gene expression in preterm neonates with FIRS was similar to that observed in systemic inflammatory response syndrome, despite known maturational differences in fetal and adult immune systems.

FIRS Beyond IL-6

Elevated concentrations of IL-6 have been used to define FIRS. However, this cytokine is simply a biomarker for the complex inflammatory reaction occurring in the fetus. Several investigators have proposed alternative biomarkers with clinically relevant correlates. Mestan and colleagues[68] used a multiplex immunoassay to measure 27 candidate biomarkers in the cord blood of preterm infants and noted that IL-1β, IL-6, and IL-8 were found to be significantly associated with the presence of FIRS, as defined by the presence of funisitis or chorionic plate vasculitis. Similar to previous studies using IL-6, these markers remained elevated even when clinical signs of intrauterine infection were absent.[64,68] CRP may serve as another potential biomarker for the presence of FIRS. Yoon and colleagues[69] demonstrated elevated umbilical cord plasma levels of CRP in fetuses with documented amniotic fluid infection and funisitis.

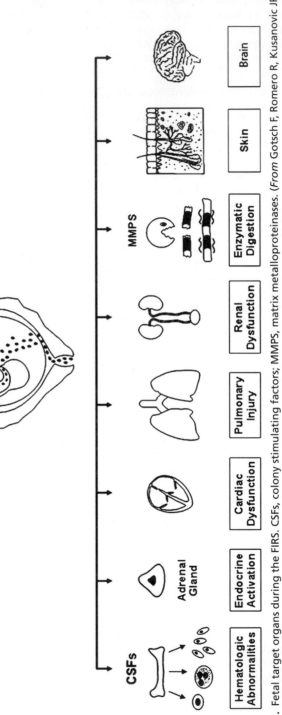
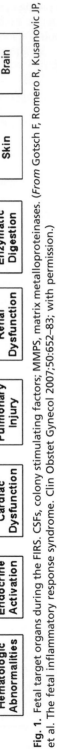

Fig. 1. Fetal target organs during the FIRS. CSFs, colony stimulating factors; MMPS, matrix metalloproteinases. (*From* Gotsch F, Romero R, Kusanovic JP, et al. The fetal inflammatory response syndrome. Clin Obstet Gynecol 2007;50:652–83; with permission.)

The specificity of CRP for the presence of funisitis was greater than that of IL-6 in this case-control study. Urinary β_2-microglobulin measured soon after birth has been proposed as another potential indicator of FIRS and was found to be associated with an increased risk for later pulmonary morbidity.[70]

The Fetal Contribution to Preterm Birth

There is evidence to suggest that the infected fetus may play a role in the onset of preterm labor.[71] The complex biochemical events involved in the initiation of parturition resemble an inflammatory reaction, with proinflammatory cytokines and prostaglandins playing a central role.[72] Romero and colleagues[73] demonstrated that the production of fetal cytokines, particularly IL-6, was associated with decreased time to delivery. Furthermore, altered hormonal signaling in the inflamed fetus results in increased cortisol production by the fetal adrenal glands, with subsequent release of prostaglandins.[42] It is though that premature parturition may represent an escape mechanism, allowing the fetus to exit the infected and inflamed intrauterine environment.[63]

Neonatal Consequences

Fetal inflammation following microbial invasion of the amniotic cavity is an adaptive host response involving the release of antimicrobial peptides, cytokines, and other inflammatory mediators. These mediators function together to combat invading microorganisms, create a barrier to further spread of the infection, and initiate the repair of damaged tissues.[63,74] These actions, designed to protect the host, are not without deleterious consequences. Numerous reports have demonstrated a significant association between fetal inflammation and the presence of neonatal brain[75–77] and lung damage.[78,79] Data suggest that the heart,[80,81] kidneys,[82] adrenal glands,[83] and even the skin[84] may be injured in the setting of FIRS (**Fig. 1**).[63]

The Altered Host

There is reason to believe that preterm infants delivered following intrauterine infection and fetal inflammation may respond differently to subsequent infectious challenges in the neonatal intensive care unit. Fetal systemic inflammation is associated with significant phenotypic and metabolic changes consistent with activation in fetal immune cells, particularly in the monocytic and neutrophilic lineages.[85] Thymic involution following chorioamnionitis has been described in human studies and animal models.[86,87] Decreased concentrations of macrophage migration inhibitory factor, a proinflammatory mediator, in the airways of preterm infants with evidence of FIRS may predispose them to pulmonary infection.[88] Future investigations exploring potential perturbations in the innate immune response of infants born following systemic inflammation in utero may reveal altered susceptibility to common neonatal pathogens.

REFERENCES

1. Knox IC Jr, Hoerner JK. The role of infection in premature rupture of the membranes. Am J Obstet Gynecol 1950;59:190–4.
2. Bobitt JR, Ledger WJ. Unrecognized amnionitis and prematurity: a preliminary report. J Reprod Med 1977;19:8–12.
3. Klebanoff MA, Regan JA, Rao AV, et al. Outcome of the Vaginal Infections and Pre-maturity Study: results of a clinical trial of erythromycin among pregnant

women colonized with group B streptococci. Am J Obstet Gynecol 1995;172: 1540–5.

4. Kenyon S, Pike K, Jones DR, et al. Childhood outcomes after prescription of anti-biotics to pregnant women with spontaneous pre-term labour: 7-year follow-up of the ORACLE II trial. Lancet 2008;372:1319–27.

5. Kenyon S, Pike K, Jones DR, et al. Childhood outcomes after prescription of anti-biotics to pregnant women with preterm rupture of the membranes: 7-year follow-up of the ORACLE I trial. Lancet 2008;372:1310–8.

6. Thorp JM Jr, Hartmann KE, Berkman ND, et al. Antibiotic therapy for the treatment of preterm labor: a review of the evidence. Am J Obstet Gynecol 2002;186: 587–92.

7. Goldenberg RL, Mwatha A, Read JS, et al. The HPTN 024 Study: the efficacy of antibiotics to prevent chorioamnionitis and preterm birth. Am J Obstet Gynecol 2006;194:650–61.

8. Ugwumadu A, Reid F, Hay P, et al. Oral clindamycin and histologic chorioamnio-nitis in women with abnormal vaginal flora. Obstet Gynecol 2006;107:863–8.

9. Gotsch F, Romero R, Erez O, et al. The preterm parturition syndrome and its implications for understanding the biology, risk assessment, diagnosis, treatment and prevention of preterm birth. J Matern Fetal Neonatal Med 2009;22(Suppl 2): 5–23.

10. Kim MJ, Romero R, Gervasi MT, et al. Widespread microbial invasion of the cho-rioamniotic membranes is a consequence and not a cause of intra-amniotic infec-tion. Lab Invest 2009;89:924–36.

11. Andrews WW, Goldenberg RL, Hauth JC. Preterm labor: emerging role of genital tract infections. Infect Agents Dis 1995;4:196–211.

12. Gibbs RS, Romero R, Hillier SL, et al. A review of premature birth and subclinical infection. Am J Obstet Gynecol 1992;166:1515–28.

13. Romero R, Sirtori M, Oyarzun E, et al. Infection and labor. V. Prevalence, micro-biology, and clinical significance of intra-amniotic infection in women with preterm labor and intact membranes. Am J Obstet Gynecol 1989;161:817–24.

14. Iams JD, Romero R, Culhane JF, et al. Primary, secondary, and tertiary interven-tions to reduce the morbidity and mortality of pre-term birth. Lancet 2008;371: 164–75.

15. Koumans EH, Kendrick JS. Preventing adverse sequelae of bacterial vagino-sis: a public health program and research agenda. Sex Transm Dis 2001;28: 292–7.

16. Koumans EH, Sternberg M, Bruce C, et al. The prevalence of bacterial vaginosis in the United States, 2001–2004; associations with symptoms, sexual behaviors, and reproductive health. Sex Transm Dis 2007;34:864–9.

17. Hillier SL, Nugent RP, Eschenbach DA, et al. Association between bacterial vag-inosis and preterm delivery of a low-birth-weight infant. The Vaginal Infections and Prematurity Study Group. N Engl J Med 1995;333:1737–42.

18. Klein LL, Gibbs RS. Use of microbial cultures and antibiotics in the prevention of infection-associated preterm birth. Am J Obstet Gynecol 2004;190:1493–502.

19. McDonald HM, Brocklehurst P, Gordon A. Antibiotics for treating bacterial vagino-sis in pregnancy. Cochrane Database Syst Rev 2007;1:CD000262.

20. Goldenberg RL, Culhane JF, Iams JD, et al. Epidemiology and causes of preterm birth. Lancet 2008;371:75–84.

21. Martius J, Eschenbach DA. The role of bacterial vaginosis as a cause of amniotic fluid infection, chorioamnionitis and prematurity–a review. Arch Gynecol Obstet 1990;247:1–13.

22. Hillier SL, Krohn MA, Cassen E, et al. The role of bacterial vaginosis and vaginal bacteria in amniotic fluid infection in women in preterm labor with intact fetal membranes. Clin Infect Dis 1995;20(Suppl 2):S276–8.
23. Andrews WW. Cervicovaginal cytokines, vaginal infection, and preterm birth. Am J Obstet Gynecol 2004;190:1179.
24. Cauci S, Culhane JF. Modulation of vaginal immune response among pregnant women with bacterial vaginosis by *Trichomonas vaginalis*, *Chlamydia trachomatis*, *Neisseria gonorrhoeae*, and yeast. Am J Obstet Gynecol 2007;196(133):e1–7.
25. Hedges SR, Barrientes F, Desmond RA, et al. Local and systemic cytokine levels in relation to changes in vaginal flora. J Infect Dis 2006;193:556–62.
26. Stencel-Gabriel K, Gabriel I, Wiczkowski A, et al. Prenatal priming of cord blood T lymphocytes by microbiota in the maternal vagina. Am J Reprod Immunol 2009; 61:246–52.
27. Schwebke JR, Rivers C, Lee J. Prevalence of gardnerella vaginalis in male sexual partners of women with and without bacterial vaginosis. Sex Transm Dis 2008;35: 78–83.
28. Josey WE, Schwebke JR. The polymicrobial hypothesis of bacterial vaginosis causation: a reassessment. Int J STD AIDS 2008;19:152–4.
29. Gardner HL, Dukes CD. Haemophilus vaginalis vaginitis: a newly defined specific infection previously classified non-specific vaginitis. Am J Obstet Gynecol 1955; 69:962–76.
30. Gelber SE, Aguilar JL, Lewis KL, et al. Functional and phylogenetic characterization of Vaginolysin, the human-specific cytolysin from Gardnerella vaginalis. J Bacteriol 2008;190:3896–903.
31. Holzman C, Leventhal JM, Qiu H, et al. Factors linked to bacterial vaginosis in nonpregnant women. Am J Public Health 2001;91:1664–70.
32. Uscher-Pines L, Hanlon AL, Nelson DB. Racial differences in bacterial vaginosis among pregnant women: the relationship between demographic and behavioral predictors and individual BV-related microorganism levels. Matern Child Health J 2009;13:512–9.
33. Simhan HN, Bodnar LM, Krohn MA. Paternal race and bacterial vaginosis during the first trimester of pregnancy. Am J Obstet Gynecol 2008;198:196.e1–4.
34. Trabert B, Misra DP. Risk factors for bacterial vaginosis during pregnancy among African American women. Am J Obstet Gynecol 2007;197:477.e1–8.
35. Bodnar LM, Krohn MA, Simhan HN. Maternal vitamin D deficiency is associated with bacterial vaginosis in the first trimester of pregnancy. J Nutr 2009;139: 1157–61.
36. Roth DE, Jones AB, Prosser C, et al. Vitamin D receptor polymorphisms and the risk of acute lower respiratory tract infection in early childhood. J Infect Dis 2008; 197:676–80.
37. Janssen R, Bont L, Siezen CL, et al. Genetic susceptibility to respiratory syncytial virus bronchiolitis is predominantly associated with innate immune genes. J Infect Dis 2007;196:826–34.
38. White JH. Vitamin D signaling, infectious diseases, and regulation of innate immunity. Infect Immun 2008;76:3837–43.
39. Wang TT, Nestel FP, Bourdeau V, et al. Cutting edge: 1,25-dihydroxyvitamin D3 is a direct inducer of antimicrobial peptide gene expression. J Immunol 2004;173: 2909–12.
40. Hansdottir S, Monick MM, Hinde SL, et al. Respiratory epithelial cells convert inactive vitamin D to its active form: potential effects on host defense. J Immunol 2008;181:7090–9.

41. Ginde AA, Liu MC, Camargo CA Jr. Demographic differences and trends of vitamin D insufficiency in the US population, 1988–2004. Arch Intern Med 2009; 169:626–32.
42. Goldenberg RL, Hauth JC, Andrews WW. Intrauterine infection and preterm delivery. N Engl J Med 2000;342:1500–7.
43. Kirschner P, Springer B, Vogel U, et al. Genotypic identification of mycobacteria by nucleic acid sequence determination: report of a 2-year experience in a clinical laboratory. J Clin Microbiol 1993;31:2882–9.
44. Lane DJ, Pace B, Olsen GJ, et al. Rapid determination of 16S ribosomal RNA sequences for phylogenetic analyses. Proc Natl Acad Sci U S A 1985;82:6955–9.
45. DiGiulio DB, Romero R, Amogan HP, et al. Microbial prevalence, diversity and abundance in amniotic fluid during preterm labor: a molecular and culture-based investigation. PLoS One 2008;3:e3056.
46. Jalava J, Mantymaa ML, Ekblad U, et al. Bacterial 16S rDNA polymerase chain reaction in the detection of intra-amniotic infection. Br J Obstet Gynaecol 1996; 103:664–9.
47. Hitti J, Riley DE, Krohn MA, et al. Broad-spectrum bacterial rDNA polymerase chain reaction assay for detecting amniotic fluid infection among women in premature labor. Clin Infect Dis 1997;24:1228–32.
48. Han YW, Shen T, Chung P, et al. Uncultivated bacteria as etiologic agents of intra-amniotic inflammation leading to preterm birth. J Clin Microbiol 2009;47:38–47.
49. Bracci R, Buonocore G. Chorioamnionitis: a risk factor for fetal and neonatal morbidity. Biol Neonate 2003;83:85–96.
50. Yoon BH, Romero R, Park JS, et al. Fetal exposure to an intra-amniotic inflammation and the development of cerebral palsy at the age of three years. Am J Obstet Gynecol 2000;182:675–81.
51. Buhimschi IA, Christner R, Buhimschi CS. Proteomic biomarker analysis of amniotic fluid for identification of intra-amniotic inflammation. BJOG 2005; 112:173–81.
52. Dudley DJ. Pre-term labor: an intra-uterine inflammatory response syndrome? J Reprod Immunol 1997;36:93–109.
53. Buhimschi CS, Weiner CP, Buhimschi IA. Proteomics, part II: the emerging role of proteomics over genomics in spontaneous preterm labor/birth. Obstet Gynecol Surv 2006;61:543–53.
54. Weinberger SR, Morris TS, Pawlak M. Recent trends in protein biochip technology. Pharmacogenomics 2000;1:395–416.
55. Buhimschi CS, Buhimschi IA, Abdel-Razeq S, et al. Proteomic biomarkers of intra-amniotic inflammation: relationship with funisitis and early-onset sepsis in the premature neonate. Pediatr Res 2007;61:318–24.
56. Buhimschi CS, Bhandari V, Hamar BD, et al. Proteomic profiling of the amniotic fluid to detect inflammation, infection, and neonatal sepsis. PLoS Med 2007;4:e18.
57. Gravett MG, Novy MJ, Rosenfeld RG, et al. Diagnosis of intra-amniotic infection by proteomic profiling and identification of novel biomarkers. JAMA 2004;292: 462–9.
58. Buhimschi CS, Rosenberg VA, Dulay AT, et al. Multidimensional system biology: genetic markers and proteomic biomarkers of adverse pregnancy outcome in preterm birth. Am J Perinatol 2008;25:175–87.
59. Di Quinzio MK, Oliva K, Holdsworth SJ, et al. Proteomic analysis and characterisation of human cervico-vaginal fluid proteins. Aust N Z J Obstet Gynaecol 2007; 47:9–15.

60. Pereira L, Reddy AP, Jacob T, et al. Identification of novel protein biomarkers of preterm birth in human cervical-vaginal fluid. J Proteome Res 2007;6: 1269–76.
61. Thompson PJ, Greenough A, Davies E, et al. Fetal C-reactive protein. Early Hum Dev 1993;32:81–5.
62. Matsuoka T, Matsubara T, Katayama K, et al. Increase of cord blood cytokine-producing T cells in intrauterine infection. Pediatr Int 2001;43:453–7.
63. Gotsch F, Romero R, Kusanovic JP, et al. The fetal inflammatory response syndrome. Clin Obstet Gynecol 2007;50:652–83.
64. Gomez R, Romero R, Ghezzi F, et al. The fetal inflammatory response syndrome. Am J Obstet Gynecol 1998;179:194–202.
65. Pacora P, Chaiworapongsa T, Maymon E, et al. Funisitis and chorionic vasculitis: the histological counterpart of the fetal inflammatory response syndrome. J Matern Fetal Neonatal Med 2002;11:18–25.
66. Redline RW. Inflammatory responses in the placenta and umbilical cord. Semin Fetal Neonatal Med 2006;11:296–301.
67. Madsen-Bouterse SA, Romero R, Tarca AL, et al. The transcriptome of the fetal inflammatory response syndrome. Am J Reprod Immunol 2010;63:73–92.
68. Mestan K, Yu Y, Thorsen P, et al. Cord blood biomarkers of the fetal inflammatory response. J Matern Fetal Neonatal Med 2009;22:379–87.
69. Yoon BH, Romero R, Shim JY, et al. C-reactive protein in umbilical cord blood: a simple and widely available clinical method to assess the risk of amniotic fluid infection and funisitis. J Matern Fetal Neonatal Med 2003;14:85–90.
70. Nishimaki S, Sato M, An H, et al. Comparison of markers for fetal inflammatory response syndrome: fetal blood interleukin-6 and neonatal urinary beta(2)-microglobulin. J Obstet Gynaecol Res 2009;35:472–6.
71. Gupta M, Mestan KK, Martin CR, et al. Impact of clinical and histologic correlates of maternal and fetal inflammatory response on gestational age in preterm births. J Matern Fetal Neonatal Med 2007;20:39–46.
72. Mohan AR, Loudon JA, Bennett PR. Molecular and biochemical mechanisms of preterm labour. Semin Fetal Neonatal Med 2004;9:437–44.
73. Romero R, Gomez R, Ghezzi F, et al. A fetal systemic inflammatory response is followed by the spontaneous onset of preterm parturition. Am J Obstet Gynecol 1998;179:186–93.
74. Janeway C. Immunobiology: the immune system in health and disease. 6th edition. New York: Garland Science; 2005.
75. Nelson KB. The epidemiology of cerebral palsy in term infants. Ment Retard Dev Disabil Res Rev 2002;8:146–50.
76. Wu YW, Colford JM Jr. Chorioamnionitis as a risk factor for cerebral palsy: a meta-analysis. JAMA 2000;284:1417–24.
77. Malaeb S, Dammann O. Fetal inflammatory response and brain injury in the preterm newborn. J Child Neurol 2009;24:1119–26.
78. Mittendorf R, Covert R, Montag AG, et al. Special relationships between fetal inflammatory response syndrome and bronchopulmonary dysplasia in neonates. J Perinat Med 2005;33:428–34.
79. Yoon BH, Romero R, Kim KS, et al. A systemic fetal inflammatory response and the development of bronchopulmonary dysplasia. Am J Obstet Gynecol 1999; 181:773–9.
80. Yanowitz TD, Jordan JA, Gilmour CH, et al. Hemodynamic disturbances in premature infants born after chorioamnionitis: association with cord blood cytokine concentrations. Pediatr Res 2002;51:310–6.

81. Romero R, Espinoza J, Goncalves LF, et al. Fetal cardiac dysfunction in preterm premature rupture of membranes. J Matern Fetal Neonatal Med 2004;16:146–57.
82. Yoon BH, Kim YA, Romero R, et al. Association of oligohydramnios in women with pre-term premature rupture of membranes with an inflammatory response in fetal, amniotic, and maternal compartments. Am J Obstet Gynecol 1999;181:784–8.
83. Yoon BH, Romero R, Jun JK, et al. An increase in fetal plasma cortisol but not dehydroepiandrosterone sulfate is followed by the onset of preterm labor in patients with pre-term premature rupture of the membranes. Am J Obstet Gynecol 1998;179:1107–14.
84. Kim YM, Romero R, Chaiworapongsa T, et al. Dermatitis as a component of the fetal inflammatory response syndrome is associated with activation of Toll-like receptors in epidermal keratinocytes. Histopathology 2006;49:506–14.
85. Kim SK, Romero R, Chaiworapongsa T, et al. Evidence of changes in the immunophenotype and metabolic characteristics (intracellular reactive oxygen radicals) of fetal, but not maternal, monocytes and granulocytes in the fetal inflammatory response syndrome. J Perinat Med 2009;37:543–52.
86. Di Naro E, Cromi A, Ghezzi F, et al. Fetal thymic involution: a sonographic marker of the fetal inflammatory response syndrome. Am J Obstet Gynecol 2006;194: 153–9.
87. Kunzmann S, Glogger K, Been JV, et al. Thymic changes after chorioamnionitis induced by intraamniotic lipopolysaccharide in fetal sheep. Am J Obstet Gynecol 2010;202(476):e1–9.
88. Thomas W, Seidenspinner S, Kawczynska-Leda N, et al. Systemic fetal inflammation and reduced concentrations of macrophage migration inhibitory factor in tracheobronchial aspirate fluid of extremely premature infants. Am J Obstet Gynecol 2008;198(64):e1–6.

Index

Note: Page numbers of article titles are in **boldface** type.

A

N-Acetyl cysteine, for meningitis, 666
Acinetobacter, in ventilator-associated pneumonia, 632
Acinetobacter anitratus, antibiotic-resistant, 553
Acute phase proteins, in late-onset neonatal sepsis, 601–602
Age, heart rate characteristics index and, 593
Amikacin, mechanism of action and resistance to, 550
Aminoglycosides, mechanism of action and resistance to, 550
Amniotic fluid
    infection of, preterm birth related to, 677–688
    swallowing of, 571
Amphotericin B, mechanism of action of, 549
Ampicillin, resistance to, 551
Amyloid, in late-onset neonatal sepsis, 601–602
Antibiotic(s)
    for meningitis, bacterial component release due to, 664
    for ventilator-associated pneumonia, 634–635
    judicious use of, 554–556
Antibiotic resistance, **547–563**
    clinical impact of, 552–554
    epidemiology of, 547–549
    in *Staphylococcus aureus,* 536–538
    mechanisms of, 549–551
    prevention of, 554–558
    to fluconazole, 617, 623–624
Apoptosis modulation, for meningitis, 665
Approximate entropy, in heart rate, 589–590
Arginine catabolic mobile element, *Staphylococcus aureus,* 538
Artificial nails, microorganisms associated with, 646–647
Aspiration, prevention of, for ventilator-associated pneumonia, 635
Autonomic nervous system, in heart rate variability regulation, 582–583, 586–587
Aztreonam, resistance to, 549

B

Bacteremia
    antibiotic-resistant, 553
    catheter-related, 648–650
    Staphylococcus aureus, 538–539
Bacterial meningitis, **655–676**
    animal models for, 656
    definition of, 655

Clin Perinatol 37 (2010) 689–698
doi:10.1016/S0095-5108(10)00089-8
0095-5108/10/$ – see front matter © 2010 Elsevier Inc. All rights reserved.

perinatology.theclinics.com

S

Moving?

Make sure your subscription moves with you!

To notify us of your new address, find your **Clinics Account Number** (located on your mailing label above your name), and contact customer service at:

Email: **journalscustomerservice-usa@elsevier.com**

800-654-2452 (subscribers in the U.S. & Canada)
314-447-8871 (subscribers outside of the U.S. & Canada)

Fax number: **314-447-8029**

Elsevier Health Sciences Division
Subscription Customer Service
3251 Riverport Lane
Maryland Heights, MO 63043

*To ensure uninterrupted delivery of your subscription, please notify us at least 4 weeks in advance of move.